INSTRUCTOR'S GUIDE

HIGH RELIABILITY ORGANIZATIONS
SECOND EDITION

A Healthcare Handbook for Patient Safety & Quality

Cynthia A. Oster, PhD, MBA, APRN, ACNS-BC, CNS-BC, ANP, FAAN
Jane S. Braaten, PhD, APRN, CNS, ANP, CPPS, CPHQ

Contributors:
Noreen Bernard, EdD, RN, NEA-BC, FAAN
Kristen A. Oster, DNP, APRN, ACNS-BC, CNOR, CNS-CP
Kathryn Palermo, MSN, RN, CMSRN

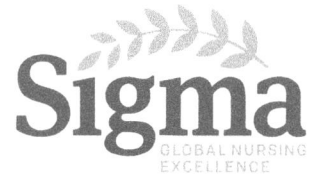

Copyright © 2021 by Sigma Theta Tau International Honor Society of Nursing

All rights reserved. This book is protected by copyright. No part of it may be reproduced, stored in a retrieval system, or transmitted in any form or by any means, electronic, mechanical, photocopying, recording, or otherwise, without written permission from the publisher. Any trademarks, service marks, design rights, or similar rights that are mentioned, used, or cited in this book are the property of their respective owners. Their use here does not imply that you may use them for a similar or any other purpose.

This book is not intended to be a substitute for the medical advice of a licensed medical professional. The author and publisher have made every effort to ensure the accuracy of the information contained within at the time of its publication and shall have no liability or responsibility to any person or entity regarding any loss or damage incurred, or alleged to have incurred, directly or indirectly, by the information contained in this book. The author and publisher make no warranties, express or implied, with respect to its content, and no warranties may be created or extended by sales representatives or written sales materials. The author and publisher have no responsibility for the consistency or accuracy of URLs and content of third-party websites referenced in this book.

Sigma Theta Tau International Honor Society of Nursing (Sigma) is a nonprofit organization whose mission is developing nurse leaders anywhere to improve healthcare everywhere. Founded in 1922, Sigma has more than 135,000 active members in over 100 countries and territories. Members include practicing nurses, instructors, researchers, policymakers, entrepreneurs, and others. Sigma's more than 540 chapters are located at more than 700 institutions of higher education throughout Armenia, Australia, Botswana, Brazil, Canada, Colombia, Croatia, England, Eswatini, Ghana, Hong Kong, Ireland, Israel, Italy, Jamaica, Japan, Jordan, Kenya, Lebanon, Malawi, Mexico, the Netherlands, Nigeria, Pakistan, Philippines, Portugal, Puerto Rico, Scotland, Singapore, South Africa, South Korea, Sweden, Taiwan, Tanzania, Thailand, the United States, and Wales. Learn more at www.sigmanursing.org.

Sigma Theta Tau International
550 West North Street
Indianapolis, IN, USA 46202

To request a review copy for course adoption, order additional books, buy in bulk, or purchase for corporate use, contact Sigma Marketplace at 888.654.4968 (US/Canada toll-free), +1.317.687.2256 (International), or solutions@sigmamarketplace.org.

To request author information, or for speaker or other media requests, contact Sigma Marketing at 888.634.7575 (US/Canada toll-free) or +1.317.634.8171 (International).

ISBN: 978164680111
PDF ISBN: 978164680128

First Printing, 2020

Publisher: Dustin Sullivan
Acquisitions Editor: Emily Hatch
Interior Design/Page Layout: Becky Batchelor

Managing Editor: Carla Hall
Copy Editor: Gill Editorial Services
Proofreader: Todd Lothery

ACKNOWLEDGMENTS

The authors wish to thank Noreen Bernard, Kristen Oster, and Kathryn Palermo for contributing their expertise and clinical experiences to make this guide relevant to both instructor and student.

ABOUT THE EDITORS

CYNTHIA A. OSTER, PHD, MBA, APRN, ACNS-BC, CNS-BC, ANP, FAAN

Cynthia A. Oster is the Patient Safety Nurse Scientist at Emory Healthcare and an adjunct Assistant Professor at the Nell Hodgson Woodruff School of Nursing at Emory University in Atlanta, Georgia. For more than a decade, Oster was a nurse scientist for Centura Health and a clinical nurse specialist for critical care and cardiovascular services at Porter Adventist Hospital in Denver, Colorado. She has held research, clinical, educational, and administrative positions throughout her 40-year career. Oster received her BSN from the University of Iowa, her MSN from the University of Nebraska Medical Center, and her PhD from the University of Colorado College of Nursing. In addition, she earned an ANP certificate from Beth El College of Nursing in Colorado Springs, Colorado, and an MBA from the University of Colorado–Denver. In 2017, she became a Fellow in the American Academy of Nursing. She mentors clinical nurses and advanced practice nurses to develop clinical practice wisdom through application of high reliability principles, evidence-based practice, and the conduct of research. Oster has presented at national and international meetings and has published in the areas of high reliability, evidence-based practice, alarm fatigue, and peer review. She is a member of Sigma Theta Tau International, the American Nurses Association, the American Association of Critical-Care Nurses, the National Association of Clinical Nurse Specialists, the American College of Healthcare Executives, and Beta Gamma Sigma.

JANE S. BRAATEN, PHD, APRN, CNS, ANP, CPPS, CPHQ

Jane S. Braaten is a Director of Quality & Patient Safety Officer and nurse scientist at Centura Health, Castle Rock Adventist Hospital in Castle Rock, Colorado. She has held positions as Director of Cardiology Services, Cardiac and Intensive Care Clinical Nurse Specialist, Cardiac Nurse Practitioner, and Manager/Charge RN/Staff RN of intensive care and telemetry units. Braaten obtained her BSN from the Indiana University School of Nursing and holds the degree of doctor of philosophy and certificates of clinical nurse specialist and adult nurse practitioner from the University of Colorado College of Nursing. She also is a certified professional in patient safety (CPPS) and a certified professional in healthcare quality (CPHQ). She has presented at national meetings and has published in the areas of hospital system barriers to rapid response team activation, quality improvement in telemetry, end-of-life care in the intensive care unit, leadership, and high reliability organizations and healthcare.

ABOUT THE CONTRIBUTORS

NOREEN BERNARD, EDD, RN, NEA-BC, FAAN

Noreen Bernard is a seasoned nurse executive with experience in leading nursing practice in acute care and ambulatory settings. She has been a leader in the areas of executive leadership, professional development, leadership development, nurse credentialing, nurse residencies, nursing practice standards, professional governance, and research. She serves as a Chief Nursing Officer in a large health system, adjunct associate professor and adjoint faculty in two academic institutions, and an administrative consultant for an academic health system. She has expertise in leadership, clinical operations, hospital construction, program development, business development, education, staffing strategy, Magnet® preparation, professional governance, regulatory readiness, and nursing practice advancement. Bernard's research is in the areas of nursing administration, resilience, job satisfaction, professional joy, and nursing practice. She earned her EdD in organizational leadership and organization development from Grand Canyon University, her master's in nursing administration at the University of Colorado, and her BSN at the University of Northern Colorado. She is Nurse Executive Advanced Board Certified and became a Fellow in the American Academy of Nursing in 2019.

KRISTEN A. OSTER, DNP, APRN, ACNS-BC, CNOR, CNS-CP

Kristen A. Oster is currently an Assistant Nurse Manager for the Operating Room at Parker Adventist Hospital in Parker, Colorado. Previously she was a Patient Safety Specialist assigned to the perioperative and ambulatory service line at the University of Colorado–Anschutz Medical Campus in Aurora, Colorado. Additionally, she has been a Perioperative Clinical Nurse Specialist and an Assistant Nurse Manager for the ENT, skull base, head/neck, and neurosurgery service line in perioperative services at Porter Adventist Hospital, Denver, Colorado. She received a bachelor of science degree in biology and education from Denison University in Granville, Ohio. Hearing the call to nursing, Kristen earned a bachelor of science degree in nursing in the accelerated program at Regis University, Denver, Colorado. She holds a master of science in nursing degree—clinical nurse specialist focus in adult and geriatric acute care and Doctorate in Nursing Practice—from the University of Colorado, Denver. Kristen is a member of the Association of periOperative Registered Nurses and Sigma Theta Tau International.

KATHRYN PALERMO, MSN, RN, CMSRN

Kathryn Palermo is currently a Clinical Nurse Coordinator for the Acute Care Unit at Castle Rock Adventist Hospital in Castle Rock, Colorado. She previously served as the Assistant Nurse Manager for Acute Care Services. Additionally, she serves as an affiliate nursing faculty member at Colorado Christian University in Lakewood, Colorado. She has developed and implemented several evidence-based practice projects addressing nurse turnover, patient satisfaction, alarm fatigue, and new graduate nurse burnout. Following the achievement of a bachelor of science degree in biology from Dallas Baptist University in Dallas, Texas, Kathryn earned a bachelor of science degree in nursing from Beth El College of Nursing in Colorado Springs, Colorado, followed by a master of science in nursing degree focused on leadership and management from Western Governor's University in Salt Lake City, Utah. She is currently pursuing a DNP degree from the University of St. Augustine for Health Sciences in St. Augustine, Florida. She is a member of Sigma Theta Tau International and the Academy for Medical-Surgical Nursing.

TABLE OF CONTENTS

UNIT 1: USING THE TEXTBOOK FOR TEACHING AND LEARNING 11

Consistency with Nursing Education Accreditation Standards *12*

Strategies for Teaching *14*

UNIT 2: RESOURCES FOR TEACHING HIGH RELIABILITY FOR PATIENT SAFETY AND QUALITY 17

Evidence-Based Practice (EBP) Resources *18*

Change Management Models *18*

Influential Resources on High Reliability Organizations (HROs) *18*

National Resources for Quality and Patient Safety *19*

UNIT 3: CHAPTER LEARNING ACTIVITIES AND INSTRUCTOR SUPPORT.. 21

PART 1: HIGH RELIABILITY: THE TIME IS NOW 22

1 THE NEED FOR A PARADIGM SHIFT IN HEALTHCARE QUALITY AND SAFETY THINKING 23

Learning Activity 1.1: Compare and Contrast External/Internal Drivers Shaping the Healthcare Quality and Safety Paradigm Shift *24*

2 CURRENT PATIENT SAFETY DRIVERS 26

Learning Activity 2.1: Differentiate Individual and System Factors Within Patient Harm Events Through Application of High Reliability Principles to Discover Solutions and Explore Barriers *26*

3 CURRENT QUALITY DRIVERS 29

Learning Activity 3.1: Discover How Evidence-Based Practice Aligns With High Reliability Principles to Inform Drivers of Quality *29*

4 ORGANIZATIONAL CULTURE AND THE JOURNEY TO HRO 33

Learning Activity 4.1: Compare and Contrast Drivers of Organizational Culture and Discuss Practical Application of High Reliability Concepts That Change Organizational Culture *33*

5 SAFETY LEADERSHIP: COMMITMENT TO HIGH RELIABILITY ORGANIZING ... 39

Learning Activity 5.1: Compare and Contrast Characteristics of Safety Leadership Styles and Safety Leadership Actions Within a High Reliability Organizing Framework *39*

PART 2: HRO CONCEPTS AND APPLICATION TO PRACTICE: PREOCCUPATION WITH FAILURE 45

6 ANTICIPATION OF FAILURE: FAILURE MODE AND EFFECTS ANALYSIS 46
Learning Activity 6.1: Discuss the Importance of the FMEA Process Within a High Reliability Organization 46

7 ACTING ON CLOSE CALLS, NEAR MISSES, AND UNSAFE CONDITIONS: THE BASIS OF HIGH RELIABILITY 50
Learning Activity 7.1: Evaluate the Importance of Near Misses, Close Calls, and Unsafe Conditions to High Reliability 51

PART 3: HRO CONCEPTS AND APPLICATION TO PRACTICE: RELUCTANCE TO SIMPLIFY 54

8 HUMAN FACTORS ENGINEERING TO ANTICIPATE AND PREVENT ERROR 55
Learning Activity 8.1: Explain Human Factors Engineering (HFE): The Science and Practice of Designing Work Systems to Fit the Needs, Limitations, and Capabilities of Humans 55

9 ROOT CAUSE ANALYSIS: A TOOL FOR HIGH RELIABILITY IN A COMPLEX ENVIRONMENT 59
Learning Activity 9.1: Discuss Use of RCA as a Tool for Embedding the High Reliability Principle "Reluctance to Simplify" Into a Safety Event Investigation 60

10 JUST CULTURE AND THE IMPACT ON HIGH RELIABILITY 63
Learning Activity 10.1: Examine the Features and Challenges of a Just Culture Within a Highly Reliable Safety Program and the Current Healthcare Environment 63

PART 4: HRO CONCEPTS AND APPLICATION TO PRACTICE: SENSITIVITY TO OPERATIONS 67

11 ALARM SAFETY: WORKING SOLUTIONS 68
Learning Activity 11.1: Appraise the Concept of Alarm Fatigue and the Possibilities for Improvement When Applying High Reliability Principles to Clinical Alarm Safety 68

12 INNOVATIVE TECHNOLOGY, STANDARDIZATION, AND THE IMPACT ON HIGH RELIABILITY 71
Learning Activity 12.1: Apply Knowledge of Effective Interventions for High Reliability to Analyze Technological Advances in Your Practice 72

13 TIERED SAFETY HUDDLES 76
Learning Activity 13.1: Describe the Value of the Tiered Huddle in Healthcare as an Effective Tool to Promote High Reliability in a Complex Organization 76

PART 5: HRO CONCEPTS AND APPLICATION TO PRACTICE: DEFERENCE TO EXPERTISE ... 79

14 INTERPROFESSIONAL COLLABORATION ... 80
Learning Activity 14.1: Describe and Explain an Interprofessional Team in the Context of High Reliability Organizations (HROs) ... 80

15 NURSES CREATE RELIABLE CARE BY ENHANCING ENGAGEMENT ... 83
Learning Activity 15.1: Compare and Contrast Assessment, Measurement, and Key Interventions to Improve Patient Experience in a Highly Reliable Organization ... 84

16 PEDIATRIC PATIENT SAFETY: UTILIZING SAFETY COACHING AS A STRATEGY TOWARD ZERO HARM ... 86
Learning Activity 16.1 Examine the Role of Safety Coaches as a Vehicle for Successful Change Management and Sustainability of HRO Principles ... 87

PART 6: HRO CONCEPTS AND APPLICATION TO PRACTICE: RESILIENCE ... 90

17 RESILIENCE: A PATH TO HRO ... 91
Learning Activity 17.1: Resilience: Comparing Personal and Organizational Resilience in the Context of High Reliability ... 91

18 DESIGNING RESILIENCE INTO THE WORK ENVIRONMENT ... 95
Learning Activity 18.1: Apply a Social-Ecological Perspective of Resilience to Support Clinician Well-Being in the Work Environment ... 95

19 BUILDING HIGH RELIABILITY THROUGH SIMULATION ... 98
Learning Activity 19.1: Explore Opportunities to Use Simulation to Improve Safety and Reliability of Risk-Prone Processes ... 98

20 BUILDING RESILIENCE THROUGH TEAM TRAINING: RAPID RESPONSE AND IN-HOSPITAL CARDIAC ARREST EVENTS ... 101
Learning Activity 20.1: Evaluate Rapid Response and In-Hospital Cardiac Arrest Event Team Performance ... 102

21 SUSTAINING THE CULTURE OF SAFETY: STRATEGIES TO MAINTAIN THE GAINS ... 105
Learning Activity 21.1: Sustaining a Culture of Safety in a Resilient Organization ... 105

PART 7: ASSIMILATION INTO PRACTICE ACROSS THE CONTINUUM ... 108

22 APPLICATION OF HRO STRATEGIES TO IMPROVE PAIN MANAGEMENT AND OPIOID SAFETY: THE CNS ROLE ... 109

Learning Activity 22.1: Examine Clinical Nurse Specialist Leadership of Clinical Improvement Teams in High Reliability Organizations ... 109

23 AMBULATORY CARE: THE FRONTIER FOR HIGH RELIABILITY ... 112

Learning Activity 23.1: Integration of High Reliability Principles to Address Quality and Safety Challenges in Ambulatory Care ... 113

24 APPLYING HIGH RELIABILITY PRINCIPLES ACROSS A LARGE HEALTHCARE SYSTEM TO REDUCE PATIENT FALLS ... 115

Learning Activity 24.1: Apply High Reliability Tenets to Solve Health System Quality and Safety Challenges ... 116

25 THE SYNTHESIS AMONG MAGNET RECOGNITION PROGRAM® MODEL COMPONENTS AND HIGH RELIABILITY ORGANIZATION PRINCIPLES ... 119

Learning Activity 25.1: Explain the Synergistic Relationship Between the Magnet Model Components and the Principles of High Reliability ... 120

26 ACHIEVING HRO: THE ROLE OF THE BEDSIDE SCIENTIST IN RESEARCH ... 123

Learning Activity 26.1: Discover the Role of the Bedside Scientist in a High Reliability Organization ... 123

PART 8: TRANSLATION INTO PRACTICE ... 128

SUMMATIVE ASSESSMENT: TRANSLATION INTO PRACTICE ... 129

SUPPLEMENTAL INSTRUCTOR RESOURCES AND READINGS ... 132

APPENDICES ... 136

INTRODUCTION

ABOUT THE INSTRUCTOR'S GUIDE

Welcome to the instructor's guide for the second edition of *High Reliability Organizations: A Healthcare Handbook for Patient Safety & Quality*. This guide is designed to be a resource for educators in a variety of academic settings in courses focused on patient safety or quality management in nursing, health services administration, or clinical programs. This instructor's guide is divided into three sections:

- **Unit 1:** Using the Textbook for Teaching and Learning
- **Unit 2:** Resources for Teaching High Reliability for Patient Safety and Quality
- **Unit 3:** Chapter Learning Activities and Instructor Support

This guide provides suggestions to guide faculty, nurse leaders, clinical staff nurses, quality and safety staff, or other healthcare professionals who are teaching others about the application of HRO principles to patient safety and quality problems using the second edition of *High Reliability Organizations: A Healthcare Handbook for Patient Safety & Quality*. For academic faculty, the chapter-by-chapter learning activities will help facilitate student learning about application of high reliability to patient safety and quality and can be used as part of a patient safety and quality course at a variety of academic levels.

The student workbook contains the same chapter-by-chapter learning activities found in the instructor's guide. The instructor's guide contains supplemental materials including learning activity implementation strategies and student evaluation sections. There are several completed examples of fill-in responses or answers for instructors as well. A summative learning activity is included that gives instructors the opportunity to assess student ability to translate high reliability principles into practice.

ABOUT THE BOOK

High Reliability Organizations: A Healthcare Handbook for Patient Safety & Quality comprehensively describes how to infuse the knowledge, skills, and attitudes of an HRO into the fabric of an organization from the boardroom to the front lines of care, including patients and their families. The book is based on the premise that although a quest for high reliability must start in the boardroom, it must also be part of every person's focus. The current message in patient safety and quality literature is that we, in healthcare, need to strive to be highly reliable, meaning that we should be a system that detects and prevents errors from happening even though we operate in high-risk, emergent conditions. Most often, the conversation goes in the direction that healthcare should be similar to aviation. This message is not helpful to healthcare providers as they strive to understand what high reliability is and looks like in the healthcare field. This book addresses that gap by providing an understanding of HRO and the application of its concepts to clinical practice. Practical examples are offered that support each of the five concepts of HRO along with useful tools, measurements, and design strategies. The various chapters tease apart the multiple facets of HROs and apply the standards to everyday components of care. Chapter content blends leadership approaches with frontline clinician application. The text places the need for high reliability concepts into our current climate in healthcare through illustrative discussion (theory and research) of each of the five concepts of HRO, along with a description of a current best practice or tool that applies to the model. The course textbook is a tool for teaching and learning. The textbook explains in Part 1 how high reliability contributes to organizational quality and safety.

It recommends in Parts 2 through 6 quality and safety activities based on high reliability principles. In Parts 7 and 8, it integrates high reliability principles into healthcare practice. Although we do not intend this as a textbook, it could be used in graduate courses focused on patient safety or quality management in nursing, health services administration, or clinical programs.

UNIT 1

USING THE TEXTBOOK FOR TEACHING AND LEARNING

CONSISTENCY WITH NURSING EDUCATION ACCREDITATION STANDARDS

Nursing faculty may use the textbook, the instructor's guide, and the student workbook to facilitate meeting of accreditation standards related to quality care and patient safety in the curriculum. The major accreditation standards relating to quality care and patient safety content follow:

- American Association of Colleges of Nursing
- National League for Nursing
- Accreditation Commission for Education in Nursing

American Association of Colleges of Nursing

The American Association of Colleges of Nursing is the driving force for innovation and excellence in academic nursing and publishes the Essentials series. The Essentials series delineates the national consensus by providing the elements and framework for building nursing curricula. The Essentials outline the necessary curriculum content and expected competencies of graduates from baccalaureate, master's, and DNP programs, as well as the clinical support needed for the full spectrum of academic nursing. These are public domain documents and are easily retrievable. Mention of quality and patient safety are found explicitly in the following:

- *The Essentials of Baccalaureate Education for Professional Nursing Practice*, October 20, 2008. Essential II: Basic Organizational and Systems Leadership for Quality Care and Patient Safety recognizes that a baccalaureate-prepared nurse must possess the knowledge and skills in leadership, quality improvement, and patient safety that are necessary to provide high-quality healthcare, including reliability and reliability sciences in healthcare. Retrieved from http://www.aacnnursing.org/portals/42/publications/baccessentials08.pdf

- *The Essentials of Master's Education in Nursing*, March 21, 2011. Essential III: Quality Improvement and Safety recognizes that a master's-prepared nurse must be articulate in the methods, tools, performance measures, and standards related to quality and safety, as well as prepared to apply quality and safety principles within an organization, including using high reliability principles. Retrieved from http://www.aacnnursing.org/portals/42/publications/mastersessentials11.pdf

- *The Essentials of Doctoral Education for Advanced Nursing Practice*, October 2006. Essential II: Organizational and Systems Leadership for Quality Improvement and Systems Thinking recognizes that organizational and systems leadership are critical for DNP graduates to improve patient and healthcare outcomes. Doctoral-level knowledge and skills in these areas ensure accountability for quality of healthcare and patient safety for populations with whom they work. Essential III: Clinical Scholarship and Analytical Methods for Evidence-Based Practice recognizes that DNP graduates engage in advanced nursing practice and provide leadership for evidence-based practice. This requires competence in knowledge application activities: the translation of research in practice, the evaluation of practice, improvement of the reliability of healthcare practice, and outcomes and participation in collaborative research. Retrieved from https://www.aacnnursing.org/Portals/42/Publications/DNPEssentials.pdf

National League for Nursing

The National League for Nursing (NLN) promotes excellence in nursing education to build a strong and diverse nursing workforce to advance the health of our nation and the global community. NLN promotes the preparation of a diverse nurse workforce that contributes to healthcare quality and safety. The NLN Commission for Nursing Education Accreditation (CNEA) demonstrates that programs meet rigorous standards that foster continuous quality improvement in nursing programs and promote excellence in nursing education. The NLN CNEA promotes excellence and integrity in nursing education globally through an accreditation process that respects the diversity of program mission, curricula, students, and faculty; emphasizes a culture of continuous quality improvement; and influences the preparation of a caring and skilled nursing workforce.

Mentions of quality and patient safety are found explicitly in the following:

- *CNEA Accreditation Standards for Nursing Education Programs*, February 2016. Mention of high reliability is not obvious; however, general reference of quality and safety is found in Standard V: Culture of Learning and Diversity—Curriculum and Evaluation Planning. A curriculum integrating "context and environment of care delivery, knowledge and science applied to implementation and evaluation of evidenced-base care, personal and professional development, quality and safety, patient-centered care, and teamwork….." is related to high reliability. Retrieved from http://www.nln.org/docs/default-source/accreditation-services/cnea-standards-final-february-201613f2bf5c78366c709642ff00005f0421.pdf?sfvrsn=12

Accreditation Commission for Education in Nursing

The Accreditation Commission for Education in Nursing (ACEN) supports the interests of nursing education, nursing practice, and the public by providing specialized accreditation for all levels of nursing education and transition-to-practice programs. The goal of the ACEN is to be a supportive partner in strengthening the quality of nursing education and transition-to-practice programs and is recognized as an accrediting body by the U.S. Department of Education and by the Council for Higher Education Accreditation.

Mention of quality and patient safety are found explicitly in the following:

- *ACEN 2017 Accreditation Manual Section III Standards and Criteria—Clinical Doctorate/DNP Specialist Certificate*, July 2020 Edit. There is no overt reference of student learning outcomes specific to high reliability, quality, and patient safety. However, curriculum standard 4.9 reflects this: "student clinical experiences and practice learning environments are evidence-based; reflect contemporary practice and nationally established patient health and safety goals; and support the achievement of the end-of-program student learning outcomes." Retrieved from https://www.acenursing.org/Resources-for-Nursing-Programs/sc2017-C.pdf

- *ACEN 2017 Accreditation Manual Section III Standards and Criteria—Master's and Post-Master's Certificate*, July 2020 Edit. There is no overt reference of student learning outcomes specific to high reliability, quality, and patient safety. However, curriculum standard 4.9 reflects this: "student clinical experiences and practice learning environments are evidence-based; reflect contemporary practice and nationally established patient health and safety goals; and support the achievement of the end-of-program student learning outcomes." Retrieved from https://www.acenursing.org/Resources-for-Nursing-Programs/sc2017-M.pdf

- *ACEN 2017 Accreditation Manual Section III Standards and Criteria—Baccalaureate*, July 2020 Edit. There is no overt reference of student learning outcomes specific to high reliability, quality, and patient safety. However, curriculum standard 4.9 reflects this: "student clinical experiences and practice learning environments are evidence-based; reflect contemporary practice and nationally established patient health and safety goals; and support the achievement of the end-of-program student learning outcomes." Retrieved from https://www.acenursing.org/Resources-for-Nursing-Programs/sc2017-B.pdf

STRATEGIES FOR TEACHING

There are several textbooks and scholarly articles on teaching strategies to facilitate the instruction and education of students. The following discussion is intended to supplement, not replace, these resources.

TEACHING STRATEGIES USEFUL IN TEACHING A HIGH RELIABILITY COURSE

Integration of real-world scenarios and student experiences into learning activities is a unique and useful teaching strategy for high reliability. Experiential learning translates high reliability concepts into reality, thus preparing the student to meet the national curriculum standards mentioned previously. Healthcare providers strive to understand what high reliability is and what it looks like in the healthcare field. Leveraging real practice situations provides accurate context for students to apply high reliability curriculum content and be able to see how high reliability can make a measurable difference in the practice environment.

STRATEGY IN THE CLASSROOM

In the physical classroom, engagement is essential. The flipped classroom (FC) supports improvement of critical thinking and problem-solving skills in students. In the FC, students learn foundational information outside of the classroom via reading assignments or watching prerecorded instructor videos. In the classroom, students engage in activities that enhance foundational information via role play, case scenarios, games, simulation, and group discussion. The goal of flipped learning is for the instructor to clarify, improve, and supplement the knowledge learned independently by students outside of the classroom and enhance problem-solving and critical thinking skills. The use of discussion boards can be useful. Discussion boards can be a beneficial platform to field questions and post announcements between classes.

STRATEGY FOR DISTANCE (ONLINE) CLASSES

The engagement of students in an online class is essential, whether the class is synchronous or asynchronous. The goal of either is to ensure students are engaged with the learning process so they perceive they are part of the learning process and, as a result, retain the material and feel engaged in the distance learning environment.

Synchronous online learning offers students instantaneous feedback, the opportunity to see their classmates, and the ability to feel more engaged in the online experience. Students are able to ask questions based on content being discussed in the classroom and can raise questions based on their own experiences or readings. Opportunities for engagement may include the following:

- Brainstorming
- Role-playing/practice
- Partner paired exercises with a large group debrief
- Small group exercises with a large group debrief
- Use of what, so what, now what learning protocol
- Appreciative inquiry
- Reflective learning with small or large group debrief
- Case study presentation
- Teach-back (peer-to-peer teaching/learning)

The advantage of synchronous learning is that students feel like talking and engage more with their peers. In addition to improved social interaction with peers, students can monitor classmates' reactions during discussions that can motivate students to continue engaging with their peers. Students appreciate receiving instantaneous feedback, are able to observe visual cues from peers, and feel a social connection in their online courses. Students feel a decrease in transactional distance. Thus, students do not necessarily need to be in the physical presence of other students to learn and feel a sense of accomplishment.

Asynchronous online learning allows students to take time to consider their thoughts, engage with the content more deeply, feel a part of the learning community, and post more reflective comments in discussion boards. Asynchronous interaction allows students to interact on their own schedule. Opportunities for engagement may include the following:

- Discussion boards for students to ask the following:
    - General questions about material/content
    - Questions about specific assignments
- Blogs or other types of posts
- Graded discussion boards as a response to an instructor-guided question
- Other kinds of technology that is supported by the online platform, such as a PowerPoint presentation, paper, or group project submission that requires peer feedback, either written or verbal/recorded

The advantage of asynchronous learning dialogue is the flexibility it provides for anytime-anywhere e-learning, which is the main convenience of online learning. Students are able to contemplate the content before responding in discussion boards, thereby increasing cognitive engagement with the content, especially if the content is perceived as difficult. Asynchronous online learning enables students the time to reflect on their own ideas as well as their peers to interact more deeply with the content.

UNIT 2

RESOURCES FOR TEACHING HIGH RELIABILITY FOR PATIENT SAFETY AND QUALITY

A variety of resources are available that can assist the instructor and enrich the student experience. Applying high reliability organization principles to clinical problems and understanding how evidence-based practice and change management methods are integrated within the umbrella of quality and safety improvement is essential. The following is a list and description of resources.

EVIDENCE-BASED PRACTICE (EBP) RESOURCES

The student and instructor need to be familiar with EBP. The student will need to be able to choose a model and apply it to a practice problem within the context of HRO. Resources include:

- Cullen, L., Hanrahan, K., Farrington, M., DeBerg, J., Kleiber, C., & Tucker, S. (2018). *Evidence-based practice in action: Comprehensive strategies, tools and tips from the University of Iowa Hospitals and Clinics*. Indianapolis, IN: Sigma Theta Tau International.
- Johns Hopkins model. https://www.hopkinsmedicine.org/evidence-based-practice/ijhn_2017_ebp.html
- JBI EBP Resources. A comprehensive toolkit for implementation of EBP. https://joannabriggs.org/ebp
- *Journal of Nursing Care Quality*. Journal recognized for application and publication of quality improvement and evidence-based practice projects as well as research. Great source for practical application examples. https://journals.lww.com/jncqjournal/pages/default.aspx

CHANGE MANAGEMENT MODELS

The student and instructor need to be familiar with change management. The student will need to be able to choose a model and apply it to a practice problem within the context of HRO. Resources include these:

- Kotter Change Management 8-Step Model. Retrieved from https://www.kotterinc.com/8-steps-process-for-leading-change/
- Small, A., Gist, D., Souza, D., Dalton, J., Magny-Normilus, C., & David, D. (2016). Using Kotter's change model for implementing bedside handoff: A quality improvement project. *Journal of Nursing Care Quality, 31*(4), 304–309. Retrieved from https://www.nursingcenter.com/journalarticle?Article_ID=3639513
- Batras, D., Duff, C., & Smith, B. (2014). Organizational change theory: Implications for health promotion practice. *Health Promotion International, 31*(1), 231–241. Retrieved from https://academic.oup.com/heapro/article/31/1/231/2355918
- Udod, S., & Wagner, J. (2018). Common change theories and application to different nursing situations. Retrieved from https://leadershipandinfluencingchangeinnursing.pressbooks.com/chapter/chapter-9-common-change-theories-and-application-to-different-nursing-situations/

INFLUENTIAL RESOURCES ON HIGH RELIABILITY ORGANIZATIONS (HROS)

Instructors will find that the seminal works of Karl Weick and Kathleen Sutcliffe provide a basis for understanding the philosophy and research that led to the HRO principles highlighted in this book.

- Weick, K., & Sutcliffe, K. (2007). *Managing the unexpected: Resilient performance in an age of uncertainty* (2nd ed.). Hoboken, NJ: Jossey-Bass.

- Weick, K., & Sutcliffe, K. (2015). *Managing the unexpected: Sustained performance in a complex world* (3rd ed.). Hoboken, NJ: Jossey-Bass.

NATIONAL RESOURCES FOR QUALITY AND PATIENT SAFETY

Students and instructors will find that a number of national resources are available to help understand quality and patient safety. Resources include the following:

AHRQ

The Association for Healthcare Research and Quality (AHRQ) is a federal agency whose mission is to improve the nation's healthcare system. The AHRQ website contains education, research, data sources, and toolkits for improvement. The AHRQ also offers funding and grants for patient safety and quality research.

https://www.ahrq.gov/

https://www.ahrq.gov/patient-safety/resources/index.html

https://www.ahrq.gov/patient-safety/education/index.html

https://www.ahrq.gov/teamstepps/instructor/index.html

ECRI and ISMP

The ECRI Institute is a nonprofit organization that focuses on safety and quality and the impact of technology. It recently acquired the Institute for Safe Medication Practices (ISMP), a national leader in proactive safety in all phases of the medication delivery process.

https://www.ecri.org/

https://www.ismp.org/newsletters

IHI

The Institute for Healthcare Improvement (IHI) website contains a plethora of resources for improving care. The site contains white papers, toolkits, education, and innovations, and it is the certifying body for the Certified Professional in Patient Safety (CPPS) credential.

http://www.ihi.org/about/Pages/default.aspx

http://www.ihi.org/Topics/PatientSafety/Pages/default.aspx

http://www.ihi.org/resources/Pages/Tools/Patient-Safety-Essentials-Toolkit.aspx

http://www.ihi.org/resources/Pages/Tools/RCA2-Improving-Root-Cause-Analyses-and-Actions-to-Prevent-Harm.aspx

http://www.ihi.org/education/cpps-certified-professional-in-patient-safety/Pages/default.aspx

NAM

The National Academy of Medicine, formally the Institute of Medicine, is an independent, evidence-based scientific advisor whose mission is to improve health for all by advancing science, accelerating health equity, and providing independent, authoritative, and trusted advice nationally and globally.

https://nam.edu/

NQF

National Quality Forum (NQF) is a nonprofit organization that specializes in data measurement and endorses and develops quality metrics.

http://www.qualityforum.org/Home.aspx

QSEN

Quality and Safety Education for Nurses (QSEN) is an institute committed to excellence in teaching quality and patient safety for nursing. The website includes toolkits, teaching aides, and research.

https://qsen.org/

TJC

The Joint Commission (TJC) is an international driver of quality and patient safety. TJC provides healthcare systems accreditation, quality and safety assessment, and improvement innovations.

https://www.jointcommission.org/

https://www.jointcommission.org/standards/national-patient-safety-goals/

UNIT 3

CHAPTER LEARNING ACTIVITIES AND INSTRUCTOR SUPPORT

Unit 3 provides chapter-by-chapter learning activities aligned with the book chapters. The same learning activities are furnished in the student workbook. In addition, Unit 3 provides instructor support. Each learning activity is followed by "Learning Activity Implementation" guidance, which includes suggestions and instructions for instructor use. The "Learning Activity Implementation" section is followed by a "Student Evaluation" section, which provides recommendations for the instructor to evaluate the student's performance on the learning activity.

PART 1

HIGH RELIABILITY: THE TIME IS NOW

Course objective: Explain how high reliability contributes to organizational quality and safety. (*analyzing*)

CHAPTER 1

THE NEED FOR A PARADIGM SHIFT IN HEALTHCARE QUALITY AND SAFETY THINKING

In this chapter, students will learn about high reliability as part of a paradigm shift in science and a social shift in thinking. Students will also learn about internal and external challenges facing healthcare and why a high reliability model is needed to address these challenges.

Chapter objective: Discuss the influence of high reliability on the paradigm shift in healthcare quality and safety thinking.

Learning Activity 1.1: Compare and Contrast External/Internal Drivers Shaping the Healthcare Quality and Safety Paradigm Shift

Learning activity objectives:

1.1 Compare external and internal drivers of quality and safety in the current healthcare system. (*analyzing*)

1.2 Discuss high reliability theory in the shifting paradigm. (*understanding*)

1.3 Explain application of high reliability theory in healthcare. (*applying*)

Prior to completion of the learning activity, the student should do the following:

- Read Chapter 1.
- Read Chassin, M. R., & Loeb, J. M. (2013). High reliability health care: Getting there from here. *The Milbank Quarterly, 91*(3), pp. 459–490.

Instructions for learning activity exercises:

1.1 Create a table for internal and external drivers. Discuss how these drivers affect quality and patient safety at both the system and the unit level.

1.2 Compare and contrast "old" thinking versus "new" thinking in quality and patient safety. Include limitations/possibilities in the discussion.

1.3 Present an article from the literature using at least one principle of high reliability in a healthcare setting. Include the following in the discussion: identify the high reliability principle, define the high reliability principle, and explain how the high reliability principle was applied in the article.

LEARNING ACTIVITY IMPLEMENTATION

Students will benefit most from the learning activity exercises working individually rather than in a group.

For Exercise 1.1, instructors should guide students to use the templates provided and direct students to be prepared to discuss how internal and external drivers affect quality and patient safety at both the system and the unit level.

External Drivers	Definition	Example	Macro Impact on Healthcare System	Micro Impact on Healthcare Facility (unit)
Regulation	Efforts to meet regulatory requirements to affect how we approach quality	Joint Commission and CMS safety and quality requirements	Affects reimbursement, certification, and functioning of the hospital system	Requires constant oversight of changing rules

Internal Drivers	Definition	Example	Macro Impact on Healthcare System	Micro Impact on Healthcare Facility
Zero harm	The internal goal to prevent serious safety events	Zero hospital-acquired infections	Need standardized tools and resources to meet this goal	Requires constant oversight and visible data

For Exercise 1.2, students should be able to distinguish between "old" versus "new" thinking and how this relates to high reliability. Mention of limitations and possibilities should be included in the discussion.

Exercise 1.3 requires students to go to the literature and find a peer-reviewed article using at least one principle of high reliability in a healthcare setting. Students should thoroughly read the article and be prepared to identify and define the high reliability principle presented as well as explain how the high reliability principle was applied.

These exercises can be accomplished in a discussion occurring in the physical classroom, in an online synchronous classroom, or in an instructor-prompted course-platform-based discussion board.

STUDENT EVALUATION

Instructors should evaluate the following:

1.1 Was the student able to give examples of current internal and external drivers that affect current healthcare organizations?

1.2 Was the student able to articulate how internal and external drivers influence our approach to quality and safety at a broad and specific level?

1.3 Was the student able to explain general characteristics of high reliability principles?

CHAPTER 2

CURRENT PATIENT SAFETY DRIVERS

In this chapter, students will learn about the emergence of high reliability organizations in healthcare as an effective strategy to redesign healthcare delivery organizations by emphasizing drivers for patient safety. Students will also learn about drivers for patient safety that relate less to the individual and more to shared accountability across the system of care.

Chapter objective: Summarize safety drivers affecting healthcare delivery systems and explore how high reliability organizations contribute to patient safety.

Learning Activity 2.1: Differentiate Individual and System Factors Within Patient Harm Events Through Application of High Reliability Principles to Discover Solutions and Explore Barriers

Learning activity objectives:

2.1 Describe the multiple layers and perspectives of patient harm in a high reliability organization. (*understanding*)

2.2 Explain the interconnection of high reliability and safety culture. (*applying*)

2.3 Appraise current solutions for improving safety in high reliability organizations. (*analyzing*)

2.4 Consider historical and current barriers to highly reliable solutions. (*evaluating*)

Prior to completion of the learning activity, the student should do the following:

- Read Chapter 2.
- View the video Josie's Story at http://www.ihi.org/education/IHIOpenSchool/resources/Pages/Activities/WhatHappenedtoJosieKing.aspx
- Consider individual and system factors that led to the error in the video *Josie's Story*.
- Read Reason, J. (2000). Human error: Models and management. *British Medical Journal, 320*(7237), pp. 768–770.

Instructions for learning activity exercises:

2.1 Define and give two example of latent and active failures that lead to patient harm.

	Definition	Examples From Your Experience
Latent failures (blunt end)	**Example:** Failure of oversight and support for new graduate nurses.	**Example:** After orientation, new nurse does not have a mentor for continued support.
Active failures (sharp end)	**Example:** New nurse makes an error due to lack of knowledge and fails to ask questions.	**Example:** Nurse makes an error in a procedure. She had never performed this procedure, did not know there was a policy, and did not know she could refuse an assignment due to lack of experience with a procedure.

2.2 Describe the Swiss cheese model of error.

Discuss latent factors and how they may contribute to error.

Discuss the impact of strong and weak barriers that allow or prevent harm.

Discuss system controls and individual controls that might strengthen barriers (block the holes in the Swiss cheese).

2.3 Find two definitions of a safety culture: Discuss solutions and barriers to achieving a safety culture based on the definitions in your current context.

Discuss two individual factors as antidotes to patient harm.

Discuss two system factors as antidotes to patient harm.

2.4 Present an adverse event (from experience or the literature) that led to harm.

Apply one principle of HRO that might have prevented the outcome.

Discuss barriers to the principle identified.

LEARNING ACTIVITY IMPLEMENTATION

Students will benefit most from the learning activity exercises working individually rather than in a group.

For Exercise 2.1, instructors should guide students to use the template provided. Instructors should direct students to be prepared to define and give two examples of latent and active failures that lead to patient harm.

For Exercise 2.2, students should be able to describe the Swiss cheese model of error in their own words. Instructors should guide students to reference latent factors from Exercise 2.1, the impact of strong and weak barriers that lead to or prevent harm along with system controls, and individual controls that might strengthen barriers (block the holes in the Swiss cheese) in their discussion.

For Exercise 2.3, instructors should direct students to the textbook and literature to find two definitions of a safety culture. Instructors should then guide students to discuss solutions and barriers to achieving a safety culture based on the safety culture definitions. These student discussions should be in the context of the student's current organization. In addition, instructors should guide student discussion to include dialogue related to both individual factors and system factors as antidotes to patient harm.

For Exercise 2.4, students present an adverse event to the class. The adverse event may be an event from either student experience or one reported in the literature. Student presentations must include application of one principle of high reliability that might have prevented the outcome along with associated barriers.

These exercises can be accomplished in a discussion occurring in the physical classroom, in an online synchronous classroom, or in an instructor-prompted course-platform-based discussion board.

STUDENT EVALUATION

Instructors should evaluate the following:

2.1 Was the student able to give examples of latent and active failures?
2.2 Was the student able to articulate how an error can occur and go through many layers of weak barriers prior to harming a patient?
2.3 Was the student able to define a safety culture and its characteristics?
2.4 Was the student able to articulate how an adverse event affects the individual and the workforce?

CHAPTER 3

CURRENT QUALITY DRIVERS

In this chapter, students will learn about current quality drivers for patient and healthcare outcomes. Students will also learn about high reliability as a framework for developing and sustaining a culture within healthcare organizations to provide care that minimizes errors and embraces current best evidence to achieve exceptional performance in quality, safety, and cost effectiveness.

Chapter objective: Explain current evidence-based quality drivers in the context of high reliability.

Learning Activity 3.1: Discover How Evidence-Based Practice Aligns With High Reliability Principles to Inform Drivers of Quality

Learning activity objectives:

3.1 Describe four key drivers of current quality indicators. (*remembering*)

3.2 Discuss the interrelationships between the drivers. (*understanding*)

3.3 Identify two key quality nursing indicators and improvement ideas based on high reliability principles. (*applying*)

Prior to completion of the learning activity, the student should do the following:

- Read Chapter 3.
- Read Makic, M. B. F., & Granger, B. B. (2019). Deimplementation in clinical practice. What are we waiting for? *AACN Advanced Critical Care, 30*(3), pp. 282–286.
- Read Oster, C. A., & Deakins, S. (2018). Practical application of high-reliability principles in healthcare to optimize quality. *Journal of Nursing Administration, 48*(1), pp. 50–55.

Instructions for learning activity exercises:

3.1 Select an evidence-based practice model from the literature or your organization. Provide a short rationale for model selection and a brief overview.

Evidence-based practice model:

Rationale for selection:

Brief overview:

Key focus/emphasis	Key concepts	Steps/stages	Strengths	Limitations

3.2 Identify one Nursing Quality Indicator and one Hospital Consumer Assessment of Healthcare Providers and Systems (HCAHPS) item. Include evidence from the literature supporting the quality indicator and HCAHPS item and a national benchmark for each.

Nursing Quality Indicator:

Indicator definition/description	Supporting evidence/sources	National benchmark/benchmark source

HCAHPS Item:		
Item definition/description	Supporting evidence/sources	National benchmark/benchmark source

    3.3 Apply the steps of an evidence-based practice model aligned with principles of high reliability to change practice.

EBP Model:	
Steps:	High reliability principle alignment:

LEARNING ACTIVITY IMPLEMENTATION

Students will benefit most from the learning activity exercises working in groups, but these exercises may be done individually as well.

For Exercise 3.1, instructors should guide students to select an evidence-based practice model used by their current organization or select a model from the literature. Students should provide a short rationale for model selection as well as a brief overview of the model that includes key focus/emphasis; key concepts; steps/stages; and strengths/limitations.

For Exercise 3.2, students select one Nursing Quality Indicator and one HCAHPS item. Instructors should guide students to retrieve evidence from the literature supporting the quality indicator and the HCAHPS item. Include a national benchmark for the quality indicator and HCAHPS item in the supporting literature.

For Exercise 3.3, instructors should direct students to apply the steps of the selected evidence-based practice model to change practice to improve patient outcomes. The students should be able to present steps for suggested practice changes in the context of the selected evidence-based practice model that show alignment with principles of high reliability.

These exercises can be accomplished in a discussion occurring in the physical classroom, in an online synchronous classroom, or in an instructor-prompted course-platform-based discussion board. Instructors may consider this exercise a graded presentation.

STUDENT EVALUATION

Instructors should evaluate the following:

3.1 Was the student able to select an evidence-based practice model? Was rationale for selection and model overview included?

3.2 Was the student able to provide evidence supporting individual selection of one Nursing Quality Indicator and one HCAHPS item? Was a national benchmark for each included?

3.3 Was the student able to apply steps for practice changes in the context of the evidence-based practice model that show alignment with principles of high reliability?

CHAPTER 4

ORGANIZATIONAL CULTURE AND THE JOURNEY TO HRO

In this chapter, students will learn about organizational culture. Students will also learn about how organizational culture can be measured and changed by leaders skilled in assessing, creating, and embedding an organizational culture that supports high reliability.

Chapter objective: Examine a large organization's culture assessment of readiness for high reliability.

Learning Activity 4.1: Compare and Contrast Drivers of Organizational Culture and Discuss Practical Application of High Reliability Concepts That Change Organizational Culture

Learning activity objectives:

4.1 Discuss the definition, drivers, and measurement of organizational culture. (*understanding*)

4.2 Examine culture in a familiar organization. (*understanding*)

4.3 Discuss examples of visible artifacts of culture within a highly reliable organization and challenges to organizational culture change. (*applying*)

4.4 Examine the features of a safety culture in a recognized organization. (*applying*)

4.5 Examine characteristics and challenges of high reliability in a familiar organization. (*analyzing*)

Prior to completion of the learning activity, the student should do the following:

- Read Chapter 4.
- Read Bellot, J. (2011). Defining and assessing organizational culture. *College of Nursing Faculty Papers & Presentations.* Paper 34. https://jdc.jefferson.edu/nursfp/34
- Read *Leading a culture of safety: A blueprint for success:* https://www.osha.gov/shpguidelines/docs/Leading_a_Culture_of_Safety-A_Blueprint_for_Success.pdf

Instructions for learning activity exercises:

4.1 Define and observe deep-seated assumptions and beliefs, espoused values, and artifacts of culture within your own organization.

- **Assumptions and beliefs:** What are the driving forces behind your organization? This could be religious affiliation, for profit, or not for profit. These assumptions and beliefs may be hidden, but they drive the values and artifacts of your culture.

My organization believes that …

- **Espoused values:** What is the written vision or mission statement of your organization?

Our vision or mission statement is written as …

- **Artifacts:** The visible manifestations of the values and beliefs of the system. This can include policies, art in the hospital, work environment, standard behaviors, expectations of leaders, reward systems, and more.

Our values are made visible by …

4.2 Discuss the application to an organization when high reliability principles are the guiding beliefs and assumptions. Brainstorm from the chapter and readings how these beliefs might be made visible to change culture.

HRO Belief and Assumption Zero Harm	Espoused Value	Visible Artifact of the Value in Everyday Practice	How Can Leaders Assist to Embed This Belief Into Culture? (practical daily actions)
Anticipation of error	Preoccupation with failure	Example: Daily safety huddle	Lead the huddle
Anticipation of error	Reluctance to simplify	Example: Just Culture algorithm	Embed the algorithm into adverse event investigation protocol
Anticipation of error	Sensitivity to operations	Example: Leader rounds on clinical areas routinely	Schedule this on calendars regularly
Containment of error	Deference to expertise	Example: Ensure that those with the most expertise are involved in decisions that affect their work	Build this practice into group charters
Containment of error	Resilience	Example: Support tools that staff may use to "stop the line" for patient safety	Publicly recognize staff members who have spoken up to avoid errors

4.3 For an online discussion:

   Does your organization measure safety culture?

   Describe the tool used and why it was chosen.

   What are the most current results?

   What is the best and lowest performing category?

   How would you go about improving the scores?

   What barriers and challenges do you see to improving scores?

4.4 Explore an organization that has been recognized nationally for being a top performer (IBM Watson's top 100 hospitals, Malcolm Baldrige National Quality Award, Thomson Reuters Top 100 Hospitals, and so on).

   Examine how a culture of safety has been established within the organization that you have selected.

   Identify three specific ways that the leadership within the organization has demonstrated a commitment to safety.

   Using the organization that you selected as a top performer, discuss how their commitment to safety has enabled and enhanced their success.

4.5 Using the worksheet that follows, assess your organization for high reliability characteristics.

Preoccupation With Failure	Yes/No
We conduct a huddle or prebriefing at the start of the shift to identify and mitigate high-risk issues.	
We always conduct a failure mode effect analysis (FMEA) before a new procedure or process is implemented to identify potential problems.	
Our rate of reported near misses or close calls is higher than our rate of reported patient events with harm.	
We publicly reward and acknowledge staff who report close calls or near misses.	
Reluctance to Simplify	
We use an analysis process such as asking "why" five times to get to the root or system causes of adverse events.	
We insist on strong interventions such as forced functions and cognitive aides to fix problems related to human factors.	
We never end an investigation satisfied with the explanation of, "It was just human error."	
Sensitivity to Operations	
We have few workarounds because our processes have been tested within the context of our work area.	
We always report equipment that is difficult to operate or understand as a safety issue.	
Policies and protocols that we need are immediately accessible, available, and easily understood.	
Our supervisors constantly observe processes to ensure that they are working as intended.	

Deference to Expertise	
When a process fails, we have the authority to correct it at the front line.	
Everyone in the hospital is encouraged to talk openly about unsafe situations.	
Resilience	
All of us stop procedures when we feel uncomfortable about a patient safety issue even if we have a busy schedule.	
We often simulate worst-case scenarios to be prepared.	
Employees who have been involved in an error share their experience openly in staff meetings to prevent recurrence.	
We receive constant assessment and training on how to deal with emergent situations.	

Scoring: One point for "Yes" and zero points for "No" responses

Score > 17 = Highly reliable

Score 10–16 = On your way to reliability

Score < 9 = Probably not as reliable as you desire

Highly reliable (Score ≥ 17): You have a strong safety culture that supports reliability by proactively identifying issues before they reach a patient. When an event occurs, you do not simplify by placing blame on individuals but instead search for system issues that led individuals toward the error-producing situation. Technological solutions and cognitive aides based on human factors science are most often employed as the best way to prevent error.

On your way to reliability (Score 10–16): Your culture is definitely on its way. You could improve by encouraging strong interventions that do not allow humans to make mistakes rather than relying on humans to reliably prevent mistakes. You realize that educating staff and working harder are most often employed as responses to error but still struggle with how to employ more rigorous means of interventions to sustain improvements.

Probably not as reliable as you desire (Score ≤ 9): Your organization could benefit from searching out opportunities for improvement through a dedicated approach to identifying near misses and close calls. This can start out as a small effort such as beginning a daily safety huddle. The huddle can ask questions that review prior events and anticipate events for the day. Transparency and actively searching out areas of risk that exist within the system that put our patients at risk is a great start.

LEARNING ACTIVITY IMPLEMENTATION

Students will benefit most from the learning activity exercises working in groups, but these exercises may be done individually as well.

For Exercise 4.1, students should thoroughly explore organizational culture and the impact on high reliability. It will be helpful to learning if students understand the concepts of organizational culture first and then apply their learning by observing their own organization.

For Exercise 4.2, students will build on Exercise 4.1 by applying high reliability principles as the cornerstone of a new culture. Students should brainstorm how they would make high reliability principles real, visible, and embedded into culture.

For Exercise 4.3, instructors should facilitate an online discussion about organizational culture, tools used to measure culture, results, and barriers/challenges to improving scores with students.

For Exercise 4.4, students will be required to go to the literature to find an organization that has been recognized nationally for being a top performer. Students should be able to discuss culture of safety, demonstrated leadership commitment to safety, and how commitment to safety enhances organizational performance.

For Exercise 4.5, students should assess their organization or an organization from their experience. Discussion of results and interventions to increase reliability can be discussed in a group or an online posting.

STUDENT EVALUATION

Instructors should evaluate the following:

4.1 Was the student able to describe how culture is created, articulated, and manifested in everyday organizational life?

4.2 Was the student able to observe and describe a familiar organization culture?

4.3 Was the student able to describe how culture might be assessed and changed?

4.4 Was the student able to describe barriers and challenges to culture change?

4.5 Was the student able to assess the organization for high reliability characteristics?

CHAPTER 5

SAFETY LEADERSHIP: COMMITMENT TO HIGH RELIABILITY ORGANIZING

In this chapter, students will learn about the vital role of leadership in creating a high reliability organization (HRO). Students will also learn about safety leadership style and associated safety leadership actions in a high reliability organizing framework to create the fearless workplace.

Chapter objective: Explain and discuss the vital role of leadership in a high reliability organization.

Learning Activity 5.1: Compare and Contrast Characteristics of Safety Leadership Styles and Safety Leadership Actions Within a High Reliability Organizing Framework

Learning activity objectives:

5.1 Describe the influence of different safety leadership styles and safety leadership actions on high reliability organizational quality and safety. (*understanding*)

5.2 Summarize high reliability organizing as a framework for high reliability safety leadership. (*understanding*)

5.3 Explain leadership strategies to build a high reliability "fearless workplace." (*applying*)

Prior to completion of the learning activity, the student should do the following:

- Read Chapter 5.
- Read Edmondson, A. (2019). *The fearless organization: Creating psychological safety in the workplace for learning, innovation, and growth*. Hoboken, NJ: Wiley.
- Consider various safety leadership styles and their influence on safety leadership actions.
- Consider the role of psychological safety in a high reliability organization.

Instructions for learning activity exercises:

5.1 Interview a local leader at your facility using the following questions and record your answers. Be prepared to share with your colleagues.

Interview Questions	Response Notes
What events in your life have had the most positive impact on your leadership and strategic thinking development? What has had the most negative impact?	
What other events, programs, or education have had the most impact on your leadership and patient safety thinking?	
What is your most important core belief that guides the way you lead?	
How do you factor in culture, diversity, or other differences into your leadership?	
How do you adapt your leadership to accommodate different age groups?	
What strategies have you used to develop a deeper sense of ownership in your followers' work and in their organization?	

How do you inspire others to achieve more than they expected?	
When you have had a significant setback at work, how did you respond? What did you learn from that setback?	
What are some of the methods you have used to foster safety thinking among peers, followers, and other leaders?	
When you look for the best candidate for a leadership role, what do you consider the most important characteristics?	

Describe the influence of their leadership style along with safety leadership actions on organizational quality and safety.

Leadership Style	Supporting Notes From Interview
Description	
Attributes	
Behaviors	
Safety leadership actions	

5.2 Go to the following link and complete the leadership assessment: https://www.mindtools.com/pages/article/leadership-style-quiz.htm

Based on your leadership style, discuss how you would use high reliability organizing as a framework for your high reliability safety leadership style. Include specific strategies for each of the five high reliability principles that may assist you as a leader to move in the direction toward high reliability.

Leadership style description:

High Reliability Organizing Framework	Leadership Strategies
Leadership preoccupation with failure	
Leadership reluctance to simplify	
Leadership sensitivity to operations	
Leadership commitment to resilience	
Leadership deference to expertise	

5.3 As a high reliability organizing leader, apply Edmondson's (2019) three-phase leadership strategy to build a fearless organization. Include psychological safety, healthy work environment, and fearless workplace in your discussion.

Leadership Strategy Phase	Leadership Strategies
Phase I: Setting the stage	Articulate how employee jobs are interdependent
	Articulate how employee jobs contribute to organizational purpose
	Reframe failure as an opportunity to learn rather than an opportunity to blame
Phase II: Inviting participation	Be crystal clear in the invitation to participate
	Demonstrate situational humility
	Practice proactive inquiry
Phase III: Responding appropriately	Express appreciation
	Destigmatize failure
	Sanction clear violations

LEARNING ACTIVITY IMPLEMENTATION

Students will benefit most from the learning activity exercises when they do them individually rather than in a group.

For Exercise 5.1, students will select a leader at their current organization to interview. Students should be able to determine their leader's leadership style following the interview and be able to discuss safety leadership style and associated safety leadership actions.

For Exercise 5.2, students should be able to discuss how high reliability organizing provides a framework for high reliability safety leadership. Instructors should guide students to include discussion about specific safety leadership strategies with real-world examples for each of the five principles of high reliability.

For Exercise 5.3, a thorough discussion of the role of psychological safety is needed. Students should complete this exercise through the lens of a high reliability organizing leader. Students should apply Edmondson's (2019) three-phase leadership strategy to build their own fearless organization, including specific leadership strategies in each phase.

These exercises can be accomplished in a discussion occurring in the physical classroom, in an online synchronous classroom, or in an instructor-prompted course-platform-based discussion board. Instructors may consider these exercises as a graded paper or presentation.

STUDENT EVALUATION

Instructors should evaluate the following:

5.1 Was the student able to describe the influence of a specific safety leadership style and safety leadership actions on high reliability organizational quality and safety?

5.2 Was the student able to review high reliability organizing as a framework for high reliability safety leadership?

5.3 Was the student able to articulate specific leadership strategies that could be applied to build a highly reliable, fearless organization?

PART 2

HRO CONCEPTS AND APPLICATION TO PRACTICE: PREOCCUPATION WITH FAILURE

Course objective: Recommend quality and safety activities based on high reliability principles. (*evaluating*)

CHAPTER 6

ANTICIPATION OF FAILURE: FAILURE MODE AND EFFECTS ANALYSIS

In this chapter, students will learn about anticipation of failure in a high reliability organization. Students will also learn about the purpose, potential uses, and challenges of completing a Failure Mode and Effects Analysis (FMEA).

Chapter objective: Explain and discuss the vital role of anticipation of failure in a high reliability organization.

Learning Activity 6.1: Discuss the Importance of the FMEA Process Within a High Reliability Organization

Learning activity objectives:

6.1 Describe the use of the FMEA as a cornerstone of high reliability. (*understanding*)

6.2 Discuss various applications of the FMEA in healthcare. (*understanding*)

6.3 Apply concepts of the FMEA to explore potential failures within practice. (*applying*)

6.4 Discuss the importance of psychological safety within an FMEA. (*applying*)

Prior to completion of the learning activity, the student should do the following:

- Read Chapter 6.
- Search the literature and find and read one article that uses FMEA as an improvement method.
- Review *Guidance for performing failure mode and effects analysis with performance improvement projects* at https://www.cms.gov/Medicare/Provider-Enrollment-and-Certification/QAPI/Downloads/GuidanceForFMEA.pdf
- Read Pidgeon, N. (2010). Systems thinking, culture of reliability and safety. *Civil Engineering and Environmental Systems*, 27(3), pp. 211–217. Retrieved from https://www.icesi.edu.co/blogs/pslunes122/files/2012/08/Systems-thinking-culture-of-reliability-and-safety1.pdf
- Think about the concept of safety imagination and how safety imagination is a key process for high reliability.

Instructions for learning activity exercises:

6.1 List at least four possible opportunities to use FMEA within your practice setting. Discuss why you believe the process is right for an FMEA, including the high-risk nature of the process and the potential for failures. Who would you involve?

6.2 Within your facility, find applications of the FMEA process and list the process examined, failures found, and solutions suggested. If your facility has not completed an FMEA, use the article as your source.

Process Examined	Main Failure Modes	Solutions Suggested	Positive Impact of the FMEA on the Process

6.3 Practice brainstorming failure modes: Select a common process and select one step in the process. List all the ways that the step could fail, the effect of the failure, and the reason for the failure.

Human failures:

- Skill-based: Lapse, slips
- Rule-based: Not following or applying a rule correctly
- Knowledge-based: Guessing when entering an unfamiliar area

System failures:

- Poor design
- Flawed equipment
- Cumbersome procedures
- Poor oversight

FAILURE MODES EXAMPLE

Process: Setting alarm to wake up in the morning on time

Step to examine: Setting your alarm

How Could This Step Fail?	What Would Happen to the Patient or System if the Step Failed?	Why Would This Step Fail? (Describe the human or system reason.)
Forget to set the alarm	You do not get up on time.	Too tired to remember
Set the alarm for PM and not AM	You do not get up on time.	Distracted; did not double-check; did not read instructions; did not know how to set the alarm and guessed incorrectly
		Setting confusing and not easily visible
Set time setting instead of alarm	You do not get up on time.	Distracted; did not double-check; did not read instructions; did not know how to set the alarm and guessed incorrectly
		Setting confusing and not easily visible

6.4 Discuss the importance of psychological safety when brainstorming failure modes within a group.

LEARNING ACTIVITY IMPLEMENTATION

Students will benefit most from the learning activity exercises working both individually and in a group.

For Exercise 6.1, students will benefit most if they can relate the use of the FMEA tool to anticipate failures. Examination of a journal article is helpful; however, discussing how the FMEA is used within the students' own practice area will be the most valuable. Instructors may consider this exercise as a graded paper.

For Exercise 6.2, students should find an application of the FMEA process at their organization. Instructors should coach students to list the process examined, failures found, and solutions suggested. If students' facilities have not completed an FMEA, the students may use the article from literature in Exercise 6.1.

For Exercise 6.3, students will benefit most working in a group to brainstorm. Brainstorming failure modes and seeking worst-case scenarios is not routine for most healthcare providers. We usually do not want to focus on how we can fail. Sharing how students' own experience with identifying failure modes in existing processes before they cause harm would be a good discussion forum.

For Exercise 6.4, students build on Exercise 6.3 to include a discussion of the importance of psychological safety when brainstorming failure modes.

These exercises can be accomplished in a discussion occurring in the physical classroom, in an online synchronous classroom, or in an instructor-prompted course-platform-based discussion board. Instructors may consider these exercises as a graded paper or a presentation.

STUDENT EVALUATION

Instructors should evaluate the following:

6.1 Was the student able to understand the relationship between use of the FMEA and anticipation of failure?

6.2 Was the student able to articulate the impact to organizational safety when an FMEA is used?

6.3 Was the student able to list opportunities for use of the FMEA?

6.4 Was the student able to apply brainstorming for failure modes within a process?

CHAPTER 7

ACTING ON CLOSE CALLS, NEAR MISSES, AND UNSAFE CONDITIONS: THE BASIS OF HIGH RELIABILITY

In this chapter, students will learn about why reporting close calls, near misses, and unsafe conditions is the best opportunity to anticipate and fix failures before harm is caused to a patient or the system.

Chapter objective: Discuss how the identification and mitigation of near misses, close calls, and unsafe conditions promotes high reliability.

Learning Activity 7.1: Evaluate the Importance of Near Misses, Close Calls, and Unsafe Conditions to High Reliability

Learning activity objectives:

7.1 Define near miss, close call, and unsafe condition. (*remembering*)

7.2 Describe the significance of workarounds. (*understanding*)

7.3 Describe normalization of deviance and the significance to safety. (*applying*)

7.4 Describe the importance of identifying near misses and close calls to improve safety. (*understanding*)

7.5 Discuss barriers to reporting and acting on near misses and close calls within the current environment. (*understanding*)

Prior to completion of the learning activity, the student should do the following:

- Read Chapter 7.
- Read Hewitt, T. A., & Chreim, S. (2015). Fix and forget or fix and report: A qualitative study of tensions at the front line of incident reporting. *BMJ Quality & Safety, 24*(5), pp. 303–310. doi.org/10.1136/bmjqs-2014-003279
- Read Paparella, S. F. (2018). First- and second-order problem solving: When rework and workarounds become an opportunity for improving safety. *Journal of Emergency Nursing, 44*(6), pp. 652–654. doi:10.1016/j.jen.2018.07.008
- Watch the video by Mike Mullane describing normalization of deviance and the *Challenger*: https://www.youtube.com/watch?v=CdTjEoqT6Mc

Instructions for learning activity exercises:

7.1 Ask three coworkers to identify a recent near miss, close call, or unsafe condition that they think might lead to patient harm in the near future.

Ask if they have reported the issue through a formal reporting system. Why or why not?

What was done to remedy the situation?

Ask if they are currently aware of "workarounds" to get things done.

Do they consider the "workaround" an issue worth reporting?

7.2 Define a workaround and significance to patient safety. Identify common workarounds and the reason they exist.

7.3 Define "normalization of deviance," and discuss how workarounds and normalization of deviance are related. In the next table, identify "normalized deviance" instances in either your personal or your professional life.

Normalized Deviance	Why Does This Exist?
Example: Driving 5 miles over the speed limit	"Police won't stop you for just 5 miles over the limit."
Example: Not scanning medications at the bedside with patient armband	"Scanner doesn't reach the patient, so we bypass"

7.4 Discuss barriers and facilitators to reporting near misses, close calls, or unsafe conditions.

7.5 Discuss three strategies to make reporting events easier and more useful to improve patient safety.

LEARNING ACTIVITY IMPLEMENTATION

Students will benefit most from the learning activity exercises working individually rather than in a group.

For Exercise 7.1, students will ask three coworkers about a recent near miss, close call, or unsafe condition. Instructors should guide students to think about how these events might lead to patient harm. Students will benefit most from this exercise if they can discuss real-life experiences of healthcare staff in identifying and reporting near misses, close calls, and unsafe situations.

For Exercise 7.2, students build on Exercise 7.1 to expand discussion to include the significance of workarounds on patient safety. The discussion regarding workarounds and the tolerance of these practices could be achieved in an online learning format.

For Exercise 7.3, students build on Exercise 7.2 to explore the concept of normalization of deviance. Instructors should guide students to link workarounds and normalization of deviance. The significance of workarounds and normalization of deviance could also be explored within a graded paper.

For Exercise 7.4, students should discuss barriers and facilitators of reporting near misses, close calls, or unsafe conditions. Instructors should guide students to discuss experiences from their organizations.

For Exercise 7.5, students build on Exercise 7.4 to discuss three strategies to mitigate barriers to make reporting events easier. Instructors should coach students to include discussion on how the strategies could be useful to staff to improve patient safety.

These exercises can be accomplished in a discussion occurring in the physical classroom, in an online synchronous classroom, or in an instructor-prompted course-platform-based discussion board. Instructors may consider these exercises as a graded paper or a presentation.

STUDENT EVALUATION

Instructors should evaluate the following:

7.1 Was the student able to discuss the value of reporting near misses and close calls?

7.2 Was the student able to identify significant near misses, close calls, unsafe conditions, and work-arounds? Was the student able to discuss how the identification of these events can improve patient safety?

7.3 Was the student able to link "normalization of deviance" and workarounds?

7.4 Was the student able to summarize barriers and facilitators of reporting near misses, close calls, and unsafe conditions?

7.5 Was the student able to discuss ways to make reporting events easier to improve patient safety?

PART 3

HRO CONCEPTS AND APPLICATION TO PRACTICE: RELUCTANCE TO SIMPLIFY

Course objective: Recommend quality and safety activities based on high reliability principles. (*evaluating*)

CHAPTER 8

HUMAN FACTORS ENGINEERING TO ANTICIPATE AND PREVENT ERROR

In this chapter, students will learn about the scope and practice of human factors engineering (HFE). Students will also learn about the value of partnering with trained HFE practitioners in their efforts to improve patient safety as well as the safety of those on the front lines of healthcare.

Chapter objective: Explore the value of human factors engineering to improve the safety of patients and clinicians.

Learning Activity 8.1: Explain Human Factors Engineering (HFE): The Science and Practice of Designing Work Systems to Fit the Needs, Limitations, and Capabilities of Humans

Learning activity objectives:

8.1 Identify error-prone processes within an organization. (*understanding*)

8.2 Develop a process map. (*applying*)

8.3 Discuss how practitioners of HFE think about work systems. (*understanding*)

8.4 Explain how the design of the work system can make it easier for errors to occur and harder to recover from. (*applying*)

8.5 Explain how practitioners of HFE approach redesigning the work system to reduce opportunities for error and to facilitate recovery from error. (*analyzing*)

Prior to completion of the learning activity, the student should do the following:

- Read Chapter 8.
- Read Holden, R. J., Carayon, P., Gurses, A. P., Hoonakker, P., Hundt, A. S., Ozok, A. A., & Rivera-Rodriguez, A. J. (2013). SEIPS 2.0: A human factors framework for studying and improving the work of healthcare professionals and patients. *Ergonomics*, *56*(11), pp. 1669–1686.
- Read Marriott, R. D. (2018). Process mapping–The foundation for effective quality improvement. *Current Problems in Pediatric and Adolescent Health Care*, *48*(7), pp. 177–181.

Instructions for learning activity exercises:

8.1 Identify an error-prone process for improvement at your organization.

8.2 Form a group to map out the current process targeted for improvement.

8.3 Identify the characteristics of work system elements (persons, tools/technology, tasks, physical environment, and organizational environment) that make it easier/harder for errors to happen. Include learning from error in your discussion.

Example: Responding to an emergent situation occurring in a negative pressure air flow room that requires responders to quickly don full personal protective equipment (PPE).

Work System Element Characteristics (persons, tools/technology, tasks, physical environment, organizational environment)	Easier for Errors to Happen? Why?	Harder for Errors to Happen? Why?	Learning From Error
Example: - Physical availability of PPE - Direction on "which" PPE should be used - Ease of "donning" PPE	If PPE is not available and has to be searched for, a delay in care will occur. If the type of PPE required for the patient is not specified, a delay will occur. If PPE is too difficult to "don," a delay in care will occur.	Ensure that a list for the PPE required is on the door of the patient room. Ensure that the required PPE is stocked outside of the room. Practice "donning" PPE in an emergent situation.	A simulation of responding to an emergent situation for a patient in an isolation room would be an example of practicing and learning from error before the error harms a patient.

Work System Element Characteristics (persons, tools/technology, tasks, physical environment, organizational environment)	Easier for Errors to Happen? Why?	Harder for Errors to Happen? Why?	Learning From Error

8.4 Brainstorm corrective actions that target/leverage these characteristics and do not rely heavily on things like training, instructions for use, and warnings to work.

Work Element Characteristic	Corrective Action

8.5 Discuss the types of human errors that most commonly occur. Give examples and a possible solution from a human factor's perspective.

Type of Error	Definition	Example	HFE Solution
Skill-based error	Lapse or slip during a frequently performed task, usually due to distraction or rushing	Entering order on the wrong patient	System does not allow for two patient charts to be open at the same time
Rule-based error	Applying the wrong rule or applying a rule incorrectly or not using a known rule	Not checking renal status prior to giving a medication that may damage kidneys	Flags in medication administration system that remind to check renal status
Knowledge-based error	Guessing and not asking for help in a situation for which the person involved has no context or experience	Patient has decreased mentation, guessing that she is just tired	Accepted triggers that mandate a call for a second opinion

LEARNING ACTIVITY IMPLEMENTATION

Students will benefit most from the learning activity exercises working in a group.

For Exercise 8.1, students should identify an error-prone process for improvement from their organization.

For Exercise 8.2, students build on Exercise 8.1 to form a group to identify an error-prone process for improvement from one group member's organization. Instructors should guide each group of students to map out the current process targeted for improvement and identify characteristics of the work system elements that make errors easier or harder to happen. Instructors should coach student groups about learning from error.

For Exercise 8.3, students brainstorm characteristics of work system elements (persons, tools/technology, tasks, physical environment, and organizational environment) that make it easier or harder for errors to happen based on their findings in Exercises 8.1 and 8.2.

For Exercise 8.4, student groups brainstorm potential corrective actions based on their findings in Exercises 8.1, 8.2, and 8.3. Students should include in their discussion human factors and ergonomics design-cycle as well as how HFEs think about work systems.

For Exercise 8.5, students should identify examples of human error from their experience to better understand the types of human errors that can occur.

These exercises can be accomplished in a discussion occurring in the physical classroom, in an online synchronous classroom, or in an instructor-prompted course-platform-based discussion board. Instructors may consider these exercises as a graded paper or presentation.

STUDENT EVALUATION

Instructors should evaluate the following:

8.1   Was the student able to discuss how HFEs think about work systems?
8.2   Was the student able to explain how the design of the work system can make it easier for errors to occur and harder to recover from?
8.3   Was the student able to explain HFE's approach to redesigning the work system to reduce opportunities for error and to facilitate recovery from error?
8.4   Was the student able to suggest potential corrective actions?
8.5   Was the student able to identify examples of different types of human error?

CHAPTER 9

ROOT CAUSE ANALYSIS: A TOOL FOR HIGH RELIABILITY IN A COMPLEX ENVIRONMENT

In this chapter, students will learn about the background, processes, and challenges of using root cause analysis (RCA) as a tool to advance safety in a high reliability organization. Students will also learn the steps in an effective RCA.

Chapter objective: Explore the challenges of using RCA as a tool to advance safety in a high reliability organization.

Learning Activity 9.1: Discuss Use of RCA as a Tool for Embedding the High Reliability Principle "Reluctance to Simplify" Into a Safety Event Investigation

Learning activity objectives:

9.1 Discuss the significance of using RCA as a tool to discover system issues. (*understanding*)

9.2 Apply the "Five Why" questioning technique to a familiar problem. (*applying*)

9.3 Discuss common problems that may lessen RCA effectiveness. (*understanding*)

9.4 Explain how bias occurs and how to avoid bias during the RCA process. (*understanding*)

Prior to completion of the learning activity, the student should do the following:

- Read Chapter 9.
- Read *RCA² Improving root cause analyses and actions to prevent harm:* https://www.med.unc.edu/ihqi/files/2018/07/RCA2-National-Patient-Safety-Foundation.pdf

Instructions for learning activity exercises:

9.1 Read the case examples regarding the errors in the first few pages of the chapter. Identify the active errors and the latent errors in the mistake.

	Active Error (human error)	**Latent Error (system issues)**
Medication error: Antibiotic given too quickly		
Ordering error: Two patients received incorrect radiology tests		
Medication error: Gave insulin instead of antibiotic		

9.2 Discuss the impact to high reliability when system issues are identified and corrected rather than correcting the individual only.

Reflect on a time in your career when an individual was blamed/disciplined for an event. How did that affect the overall culture of safety?

Did the error recur?

9.3 Identify a safety issue:

Practice asking "Five Whys" to get to the root cause.

The first "why" addresses the one most proximate to the error, usually a clinician. The last "why" question should be at the system level.

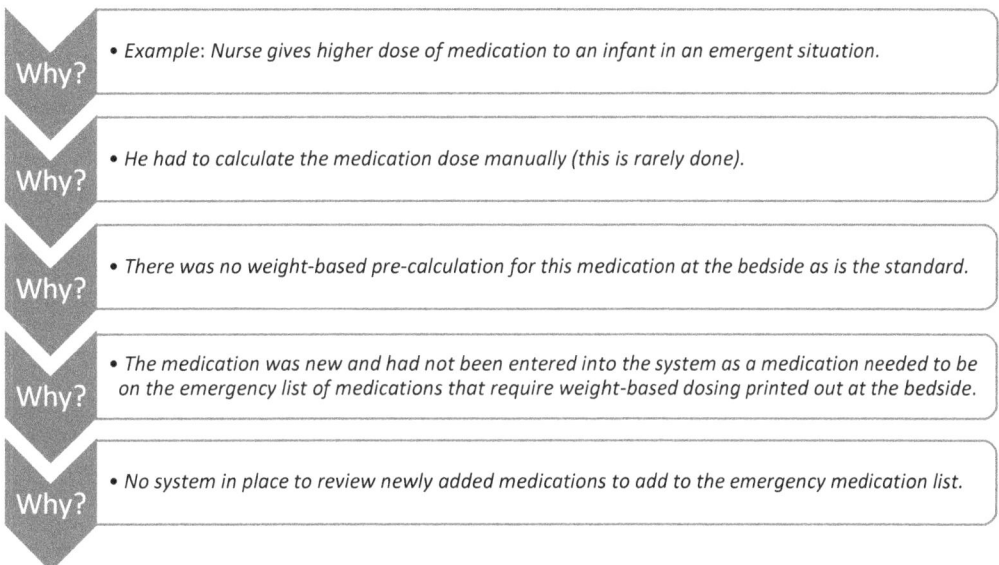

9.4 List three strategies to ensure RCA is effective to prevent future error.

LEARNING ACTIVITY IMPLEMENTATION

Students will benefit most from the learning activity exercises working either individually or in a group.

For Exercise 9.1, students should read and reflect on the science and philosophy behind the RCA and the relevance to the HRO principle of reluctance to simplify. Instructors should guide discussion of the case examples to distinguish between the symptoms of a problem (active failures) and the root causes of a problem (latent failures). Instructors can use the Swiss cheese model to illustrate the difference between the two types of failures.

For Exercise 9.2, students should reflect on the impact to high reliability when system issues are identified and corrected rather than correcting only the individual. Instructors should guide discussion to include the impact of blame on the culture of safety.

For Exercise 9.3, students practice asking the "Five Whys" to identify the root cause of an occurrence. Instructors should guide students to begin with the first "why" most proximate to the error and finish with a fifth "why" at the system level.

For Exercise 9.4, students list strategies to ensure RCA is effective. Instructors should guide students to refer to the RCA² reading. The reading lists specific skills needed for an RCA and factors that make an RCA less effective. Students may reflect on this reading and discuss RCAs that did not make an impact and those that did. Discussion surrounding the strength of interventions used within an RCA may also be effective to learning.

These exercises can be accomplished in a discussion occurring in the physical classroom, in an online synchronous classroom, or in an instructor-prompted course-platform-based discussion board. Instructors may consider these exercises as a graded paper or a presentation.

STUDENT EVALUATION

Instructors should evaluate the following:

9.1 Was the student able to articulate the difference between active and latent factors and give examples of both?

9.2 Was the student able to distinguish the significance of digging deeper than the manifest symptoms of a safety problem?

9.3 Was the student able to discuss how RCAs can be made more effective?

9.4 Was the student able to practice asking "Why" until getting to a root cause?

CHAPTER

10

JUST CULTURE AND THE IMPACT ON HIGH RELIABILITY

In this chapter, students will learn about Just Culture. Students will also learn about the challenges of Just Culture in practice due to outcome bias, misapplication of the assumptions, and application of the Just Culture algorithm without a clear commitment to the tenets of the culture change needed to learn from errors.

Chapter objective: Discover the history, theory, and challenges of implementing Just Culture in practice.

Learning Activity 10.1: Examine the Features and Challenges of a Just Culture Within a Highly Reliable Safety Program and the Current Healthcare Environment

Learning activity objectives:

10.1 Compare and contrast a Just Culture versus a blameless culture versus a punitive culture. (*analyzing*)

10.2 Apply Just Culture principles to examples. (*applying*)

10.3 Discuss the impact of second victim syndrome. (*understanding*)

10.4 Describe the differences between a retributive Just Culture and a restorative Just Culture. (*understanding*)

10.5 Discuss challenges to a Just Culture. (*understanding*)

Prior to completion of the learning activity, the student should do the following:

- Read Chapter 10.

- Watch the video *Annie's Story*: https://youtu.be/zeldVu-3DpM

- Find and read an article on second victim syndrome. Option: Ozeke, O., Ozeke, V., Coskun, O., & Budakoglu, I. I. (2019). Second victims in health care: Current perspectives. *Advances in Medical Education and Practice*, *10*, pp. 593–603. Retrieved from https://doi.org/10.2147/AMEP.S185912

- Read the *Restorative Just Culture checklist:* https://safetydifferently.com/restorative-just-culture-checklist/restorativejustculturechecklist-2/

- Read *Reckless homicide at Vanderbilt? A Just Culture analysis:* https://www.linkedin.com/pulse/reckless-homicide-vanderbilt-just-culture-analysis-david-marx/

Instructions for learning activity exercises:

10.1 Discuss the differences between a blameless culture, a punitive culture, and a Just Culture and the effects to patient safety for each type of culture.

10.2 Define the three types of errors that can occur, and give examples from your experience.

Type of Error	Definition	Example in Practice	How Is This Normally Dealt With?	How Could It Be Dealt With to Promote a Just Culture?
Human error	Example: Slips, lapses. Not intentional. Usually related to distraction.	Getting called out of a room for an emergency and forgetting to set the bed alarm for a high-risk fall patient.		
Risky behavior	Not following a rule without realizing the significance to safety.	Not turning on a bed alarm for a high-risk fall patient because the family said they would watch the patient.		
Reckless behavior	Not following a rule without regard for the significance to safety.	Not turning on a bed alarm for a high-risk fall patient because the staff member is "tired of hearing the alarm."		

10.3 Interview a manager within your organization. Find the following:
- Current Just Culture algorithm used in the facility
- How the manager was trained to use the algorithm
- Example of how the algorithm has been used to promote positive learning
- If there is a second victim program or a support system for those involved in errors
- Any difficulties in applying the Just Culture process, especially when the outcome of the error was serious

10.4 Discuss the impact of involvement in an error with the healthcare provider.

Describe second victim syndrome and the effect on the individual and the healthcare system.

Discuss how a restorative Just Culture can assist in healing the individual involved in the error and can affect system safety and healing.

10.5 Discuss challenges to Just Culture and outcome bias when the outcome is catastrophic.

Reflect on the Vanderbilt case above or another case involving litigation or media coverage.

How does the outcome bias affect the application of Just Culture?

CASE STUDY

The hospital has a new program aimed at reducing surgical site infections. The responsibility for administering antibiotics has been put in the hands of the anesthesia provider in the operating room to guarantee infusion within one hour of incision. If the patient needs a special antibiotic protocol requiring more than one antibiotic, the process is started in the pre-op area.

Kathy is an experienced pre-op nurse. A full schedule coupled with a sick call has made for a busy morning. In reviewing the schedule and her assignment, she sees that Mr. Wright is scheduled for a new procedure and will need three antibiotics before surgery. After her initial assessment, Kathy hangs the first antibiotic, Vancomycin 1 GM, and signs the medication administration sheet. She returns in 90 minutes and hangs the second antibiotic, Gentamycin 80 mg.

The CRNA who is new to the service stops in the pre-op area to read the chart of the patient. The CRNA takes the paper record to the conference room. Kathy returns to the bedside and checks her order on the CPOE for the final antibiotic and hangs the Ancef, 1 GM. The paper MAR is with the chart, so she makes a mental note to sign the MAR before the patient goes to the OR. The antibiotic infusion is finished, but Kathy forgets to go back to the chart because her usual practice is to sign the MAR when she hangs the medication.

An orderly comes to pick up the patient for the OR. Upon entering the OR, the CRNA notices that two of the three antibiotics have been administered and proceeds to hang Ancef prior to the procedure. The patient receives the duplicate dose before the presurgical nurse (Kathy) remembers she did not sign the MAR and calls into the room. The patient had no adverse outcome.

Questions for Discussion

1. Is this error an example of human error, negligence, recklessness, or an intentional rule violation? Support your answer with your rationale.

2. How should the unit manager approach Kathy when beginning her investigation into the situation?
3. What type of investigation would be the most effective in this situation?
4. What type of action is warranted based on the type of behavior that was displayed?

LEARNING ACTIVITY IMPLEMENTATION

Students will benefit most from the learning activity exercises working individually.

For Exercise 10.1, students should be able to differentiate blameless culture, punitive culture, and Just Culture. In addition, instructors should coach students to discuss the effects of each type of culture to patient safety.

For Exercise 10.2, students should provide examples of the three types of error from practice. Instructors should be mindful that examples from practice are helpful to understand the specific behaviors that are looked at within an error.

For Exercise 10.3, instructors may facilitate student discussion to compare different types of Just Culture algorithms and associated variations in practice.

For Exercise 10.4, instructors should facilitate discussion about the impact of involvement in an error on a healthcare provider. Discussion should include second victim syndrome and restorative Just Culture. This exercise could be a short graded paper with sources of evidence.

For Exercise 10.5, instructors should facilitate student reflection discussion on the Vanderbilt Just Culture analysis case. The role of media coverage, litigation, and outcome bias should also be included in the discussion.

The case study is optional and can be used as an online posting.

These exercises can be accomplished in a discussion occurring in the physical classroom, in an online synchronous classroom, or in an instructor-prompted course-platform-based discussion board.

STUDENT EVALUATION

Instructors should evaluate the following:

10.1 Was the student able to articulate the main principles of Just Culture in theory?

10.2 Was the student able to apply these principles in current practice and give examples?

10.3 Was the student able to articulate the impact of second victim syndrome and relate a restorative Just Culture to this syndrome?

10.4 Was the student able to discuss challenges to Just Culture, particularly outcome bias?

10.5 Was the student able to discuss Just Culture and the principles of high reliability in the context of the case study?

PART 4

HRO CONCEPTS AND APPLICATION TO PRACTICE: SENSITIVITY TO OPERATIONS

Course objective: Recommend quality and safety activities based on high reliability principles. (*evaluating*)

CHAPTER 11

ALARM SAFETY: WORKING SOLUTIONS

In this chapter, students will learn about improvements directed toward alarm safety in response to harm related to alarm fatigue, increased technology, and regulatory guidance. Students will also learn about interventions based on high reliability principles as a strategy for sustainable alarm safety.

Chapter objective: Explore the high-risk nature of clinical alarm management and the challenges of identifying and containing the risk to prevent adverse events.

Learning Activity 11.1: Appraise the Concept of Alarm Fatigue and the Possibilities for Improvement When Applying High Reliability Principles to Clinical Alarm Safety

Learning activity objectives:

11.1 Consider the implications of alarm fatigue within the clinical environment. (*understanding*)

11.2 Apply concepts of failure mode effects analysis (FMEA) to appraise clinical alarms within a practice environment. (*applying*)

Prior to completion of the learning activity, the student should do the following:

- Read Chapter 11.
- Read *Alarm fatigue: A concept analysis:* https://www.himss.org/resources/alarm-fatigue-concept-analysis
- Read Hravnak, M., Pellathy, T., Chen, L., Dubrawski, A., Wertz, A., Clermont, G., & Pinsky, M. R. (2018). A call to alarms: Current state and future directions in the battle against alarm fatigue. *Journal of Electrocardiology, 51*(6S), pp. S44–S48. https://www.ncbi.nlm.nih.gov/pmc/articles/PMC6263784/pdf/nihms-1502834.pdf

Instructions for learning activity exercises:

11.1 Define alarm fatigue, give examples, and discuss the implications for patient safety and high reliability.

Include examples of actionable versus nonactionable alarms and the implication for alarm fatigue.

Describe how healthcare organizations are improving the safety of clinical alarms.

Discuss how these organizations used data to track progress.

Finally, discuss how high reliability principles and improvement concepts were used in the improvement efforts.

- Include preoccupation with failure, attention to detail, and deference to expertise.
- Include standardization and situational awareness.

11.2 Perform an assessment of clinical alarms or noise distraction in your area of experience within a failure mode effect analysis format (FMEA).

Alarm	Expected Response	How Could Response Fail?	What Would Happen to a Patient Due to a Failure?	Why Would This Response Fail?
Example: Low or high heart rate alarm	Clinical goes to room and checks patient immediately	Clinician does not hear alarm or is not alerted to alarm	Mortality/morbidity	Alarm volume not checked
		Clinician is in another room		No alert system
		Clinician thinks the alarm is not "real" due to frequency of false alarms		Alarm fatigue

Alarm	Expected Response	How Could Response Fail?	What Would Happen to a Patient Due to a Failure?	Why Would This Response Fail?

LEARNING ACTIVITY IMPLEMENTATION

Students will benefit the most from the learning activity exercises working individually.

For Exercise 11.1, instructors should guide students to define alarm fatigue, give examples, and discuss the implications for patient safety and high reliability. Students should be encouraged to go to the literature to find evidence in support of definitions and examples. This exercise could be completed as a short graded paper with references from current literature.

For Exercise 11.2, students integrate the FMEA process into alarm assessment and safety. Students can refer to Chapter 6 in the textbook for a template or use the table provided. Students who are not in an environment with clinical alarms can interview a colleague who works in the environment or visit a department with clinical alarms to assess the impact of alarms.

These exercises can be accomplished in a discussion occurring in the physical classroom, in an online synchronous classroom, or in an instructor-prompted course-platform-based discussion board.

STUDENT EVALUATION

Instructors should evaluate the following:

11.1 Was the student able to articulate the definition and implications of alarm fatigue?

11.2 Was the student able to apply knowledge gained from reading to identify sources of and potential failure modes of clinical alarms?

CHAPTER 12

INNOVATIVE TECHNOLOGY, STANDARDIZATION, AND THE IMPACT ON HIGH RELIABILITY

In this chapter, students will learn how new and innovative technology, automation, standardization, and forcing functions are effective approaches to making a process highly reliable. Students will also learn that successful integration of technologies requires a systematic approach, an understanding of the learning health system, and a commitment to patient safety as a foundational value to achieve highly reliable performance.

Chapter objective: Examine how technology can be used to effectively hardwire processes and improve results.

Learning Activity 12.1: Apply Knowledge of Effective Interventions for High Reliability to Analyze Technological Advances in Your Practice

Learning activity objectives:

12.1 Discuss technology and its impact on high reliability in your environment. (*understanding*)

12.2 Analyze current safety interventions from your experience and place them in the Institute for Safe Medication Practices (ISMP) hierarchy of interventions. (*analyzing*)

12.3 Discuss the significance of workarounds, including why workarounds occur and how to mitigate them. (*understanding*)

Prior to completion of the learning activity, the student should do the following:

- Read Chapter 12.
- Read *Education is "predictably disappointing" and should never be relied upon alone to improve safety* at https://www.ismp.org/resources/education-predictably-disappointing-and-should-never-be-relied-upon-alone-improve-safety
- Read *Human factors engineering* at https://psnet.ahrq.gov/primer/human-factors-engineering

Instructions for learning activity exercises:

12.1 Assess your work environment. List examples of how technology is used and what impact it has on patient safety and high reliability. Consider the following in the discussion:

 How does the technology improve workflow?

 How does the technology improve communication?

 How does the technology improve patient safety?

 Do end users see the value of the technology?

 Are there any unexpected consequences that were found after implementation?

12.2 Use the ISMP hierarchy and list examples of each level of the hierarchy in relation to your practice and prevention of high-risk events. List the pros and cons and safety effectiveness of each level.

Risk-Reduction Strategy	Example in Practice	Pros	Cons	How Does This Improve Individual Safety?	How Does This Improve System Safety?	Will This Prevent the Error From Recurring?
Education and information						
Rules and policies						
Checklists and double-check systems						
Standardization and protocols						
Automation and computerization						
Forcing functions and constraints						

12.3 The goal of high reliability strategies is to make it easier to do the right thing and harder to do the wrong thing. Workarounds are commonly created because it is difficult to do the right thing. Discuss workarounds to various practices, why they were created, and how to mitigate them. An example is given.

Safety Technology	Workaround	Why Does It Exist?	How Can It Be Fixed?
Bedside scanning of medications	Lack of scanning at bedside	Scanner doesn't reach the bedside and is attached to the computer	Wireless scanner

LEARNING ACTIVITY IMPLEMENTATION

Students will benefit the most from these exercises by doing them individually rather than in a group. The exercises are best completed with students applying the knowledge learned to their own experience.

For Exercise 12.1, students should assess their work environment. They should list examples of how technology is used and how it affects patient safety and high reliability. If any students do not have a practice environment, encourage them to interview a clinician in their field of interest to obtain the work environment examples.

For Exercise 12.2, students use the ISMP hierarchy and table template. Students should list examples of each level of the hierarchy in relation to their practice and prevention of high-risk events. Instructors should remind students to include a list of the pros and cons and safety effectiveness of each level.

For Exercise 12.3, instructors should focus students on workarounds. They should encourage students to discuss workarounds to various practices in their practice environment. Instructors should coach students to include why workarounds are created and how workarounds can be mitigated.

These exercises can be accomplished in a discussion occurring in the physical classroom, in an online synchronous classroom, or in an instructor-prompted course-platform-based discussion board. A short graded paper with references discussing technology, pros and cons, effect on patient safety, and inherent workarounds is an option.

STUDENT EVALUATION

Instructors should evaluate the following:

12.1 Was the student able to evaluate current technology in their practice and the impact (or not) on safety and reliability?

12.2 Was the student able to articulate how the ISMP hierarchy of interventions relates to high reliability?

12.3 Was the student able to articulate the meaning of workarounds and why they are created?

CHAPTER 13

TIERED SAFETY HUDDLES

In this chapter, students will learn about the concept of a tiered safety huddle as a strategy to maintain an awareness of operational conditions in a high reliability organization. Students will also learn about how tiered safety huddles used to ensure problems from the front line of care are escalated to higher levels within the organization for awareness, system accountability, and resolution of the problem.

Chapter objective: Examine the tiered safety huddle as a vehicle to increase organization and system situational awareness.

Learning Activity 13.1: Describe the Value of the Tiered Huddle in Healthcare as an Effective Tool to Promote High Reliability in a Complex Organization

Learning activity objectives:

13.1 Describe the purpose and the value of a tiered huddle to patient safety and quality. (*understanding*)

13.2 Examine how a tiered huddle contributes to the principles of high reliability within a complex healthcare environment. (*applying*)

Prior to completion of the learning activity, the student should do the following:

- Read Chapter 13.
- Visit Today's Hospitalist website: https://www.todayshospitalist.com/tiered-safety-huddles-target-zero-harm/
- Read World Health Organization Course 3: https://www.who.int/patientsafety/education/curriculum/course3_handout.pdf

Instructions for learning activity exercises:

13.1 Assess your current work environment or interview a clinician in a healthcare work environment. Ask:

Questions	Response Notes
How are problems surfaced by those at the front line of care?	
How often do those from the front line bring up issues?	
Is there a formal mechanism to ensure these issues are recorded and escalated to those who can resolve the problems?	
Are your senior leaders aware of the daily challenges at the front line of care?	
Are they made aware of these challenges on a daily basis?	
What is the senior leader's role and response to resolve daily challenges?	
How does the resolution make it back to the front line?	
How do issues that involve the "system"—such as complex processes and procedures, equipment issues, and contract issues—get resolved?	
How are problems surfaced by those at the front line of care?	
How often do those from the front line bring up issues?	

13.2 Search the literature to consider healthcare as a complex system. Discuss the following:

Define a complex system.

List characteristics of healthcare systems that contribute to complexity.

Discuss how a tiered huddle contributes to all principles of high reliability.

How does a tiered huddle provide a mechanism to handle aspects of complexity?

LEARNING ACTIVITY IMPLEMENTATION

Students will benefit most from these exercises when they do them individually rather than in a group.

Exercise 13.1 can be completed as a structured classroom discussion or as an online discussion. The objective is to assess how frontline issues are escalated or not escalated within the student's organization to explain the value of the tiered huddle.

Exercise 13.2 can be completed as a graded paper with references or as an online posting. The purpose is to understand complexity in healthcare, connect high reliability principles, and connect the tiered huddle as an effective intervention in a complex environment.

These exercises can be accomplished in a discussion occurring in the physical classroom, in an online synchronous classroom, or in an instructor-prompted course-platform-based discussion board. A short graded paper with references is an option.

STUDENT EVALUATION

Instructors should evaluate the following:

13.1 Was the student able to describe the characteristics and the purpose of the tiered huddle?

13.2 Was the student able to articulate the value of the tiered huddle as a vehicle to promote high reliability principles within a complex healthcare environment?

PART 5

HRO CONCEPTS AND APPLICATION TO PRACTICE: DEFERENCE TO EXPERTISE

Course objective: Recommend quality and safety activities based on high reliability principles. (*evaluating*)

CHAPTER 14

INTERPROFESSIONAL COLLABORATION

In this chapter, students will learn about how an increased focus on quality, safety, and efficiency in healthcare has placed greater attention on understanding the complexity of healthcare teams. Students will also learn about interprofessional collaboration and teamwork in the context of high reliability organizations (HROs).

Chapter objective: Illustrate interprofessional collaboration and teamwork in the context of high reliability organizations (HROs).

Learning Activity 14.1: Describe and Explain an Interprofessional Team in the Context of High Reliability Organizations (HROs)

Learning activity objectives:

14.1 Describe interprofessional collaboration in the context of high reliability organizations. (*understanding*)

14.2 Explain teamwork in the context of high reliability organizations. (*applying*)

Prior to completion of the learning activity, the student should do the following:

- Read Chapter 14.
- Read Rosen, M. A., DiazGranados, D., Dietz, A. S., Benishe, L. E., Pronovost, P. J., & Weaver, S. J. (2018). Teamwork in healthcare: Key discoveries enabling safer, high quality care. *American Psychologist*, 73(4), pp. 433–450.
- Consider characteristics of effective interprofessional teams.
- Consider evidence-based tools that support teams in assessing the current state to best identify short-term goals for improving team function.

Instructions for learning activity exercises:

14.1 Describe the characteristics of an interprofessional collaborative team in your organization. Include an assessment of the strengths and weaknesses of the team using one evidence-based tool.

Interprofessional Team Name: CAUTI Prevention Team

Team characteristics

Characteristic	Description
Team leadership	Clear, common purpose
	Clear role definition for each member
	Work assigned thoughtfully to content expert
	Members involved in decision-making
Trust	Team members able to voice disagreements without fear of retaliation
	Conflict effectively managed
Backup behavior	Team decision-making process tries to make efficacious recommendations for all patients

Team assessment

Evidence-based assessment tool: Team Decision-Making Questionnaire (TDMQ)

Strengths	Weaknesses
Conflict effectively managed	Clinical staff's perception of decision-making
Trust	Shared mental model

14.2 Based on your assessment, make recommendations on how to strengthen the performance of the interprofessional collaborative team in the context of a high reliability organization. Include one team training strategy and rationale for use.

Weakness	Recommendation for Improvement (include team training strategy with rationale)	High Reliability Context (link to high reliability principles)
Clinical staff's perception of decision-making	TeamSTEPPS training to facilitate development of a shared mental model and development of continuous team communication to improve staff's perception of decision-making	Commitment to resilience

LEARNING ACTIVITY IMPLEMENTATION

Students will benefit most from these learning activities when an interprofessional team at the student organization is used for the learning activities. Optimally, the student should be a member of the interprofessional team.

For Exercise 14.1, students assess strengths and weaknesses of an interprofessional team using one of the evidence-based tools presented in the chapter. Students must include characteristics of effective teams in the discussion.

For Exercise 14.2, students make recommendations to strengthen the interprofessional team based on the assessment completed in Learning Activity 14.1. Recommendations must include one team training strategy along with rationale for use. In addition, students should include linking team characteristics to high reliability in the discussion.

These exercises can be accomplished in a discussion occurring in the physical classroom, in an online synchronous classroom, or in an instructor-prompted course-platform-based discussion board. Also, instructors may consider this exercise as a graded paper or student presentation to the class.

STUDENT EVALUATION

Instructors should evaluate the following:

14.1 Was the student able to identify and describe the characteristics of an interprofessional team? Was the assessment of team strengths and weaknesses completed using an evidence-based tool?

14.2 Was the student able to make recommendations to improve team performance that included one team training strategy? Was the student able to link effective team characteristics and high reliability principles?

CHAPTER 15

NURSES CREATE RELIABLE CARE BY ENHANCING ENGAGEMENT

In this chapter, students will learn about healthcare organizations' focus on improving the patient experience given public data reporting, pay for performance, consumer awareness and demand for value, and the tightly coupled relationships between patient experience, patient safety, and quality of care. Students will also learn about drivers and measurements of patient experience and partnering with patients to understand patient needs.

Chapter objective: Explore how partnership and collaboration with patients contributes to the achievement of a consistent, highly reliable patient experience.

Learning Activity 15.1: Compare and Contrast Assessment, Measurement, and Key Interventions to Improve Patient Experience in a Highly Reliable Organization

Learning activity objectives:

15.1 Examine how patient experience is measured and the importance and effect of measurement. (*applying*)

15.2 Appraise and examine hospital systems public patient experience measures. (*applying*)

15.3 Evaluate the current Hospital Consumer Assessment of Healthcare Providers and Systems (HCAHPS). (*understanding*)

15.4 Analyze various patient experience improvement practices and discuss the reliability of these efforts to achieve and sustain a positive patient experience. (*analyzing*)

Prior to completion of the learning activity, the student should do the following:

- Read Chapter 15.
- Visit CMS.gov to explore HCAHPS: https://www.cms.gov/Medicare/Quality-Initiatives-Patient-Assessment-Instruments/HospitalQualityInits/HospitalHCAHPS
- Visit and explore the Hospital Compare website: https://www.medicare.gov/hospitalcompare/search.html

Instructions for learning activity exercises:

15.1 Describe how patient experience is measured and improved within your practice environment, or interview a clinician within a practice environment.

15.2 Visit and compare three hospitals within your state on the Hospital Compare website.

Which hospital scores highest in patient experience?

Which category of score is the highest? Lowest?

How does public reporting affect consumer choice?

How does this affect hospital finances?

15.3 Discuss the Hospital Consumer Assessment of Healthcare Providers and Systems (HCAHPS).

How is this survey used to measure patient experience?

Is this a reliable and valid tool for measurement?

What are the challenges in measurement of patient experience with this tool?

15.4 Discuss how standardization of the patient experience occurs in a highly reliable organization.

Search the literature for examples of patient experience tools that have been successfully standardized and are considered industry best practices.

Discuss how patients were involved in creating these tools.

Describe how these practices ensure high reliability.

LEARNING ACTIVITY IMPLEMENTATION

Students will benefit most from these learning activities when they do them individually rather than in a group.

For Exercise 15.1, students should be able to describe how patient experience is measured and improved within their practice environment or interview a clinician within a practice environment.

For Exercise 15.2, students visit the Hospital Compare website, compare three hospitals in their home state, and discuss their findings. Exercise 15.2 builds on Exercise 15.1. Instructors should facilitate student discussion to connect Hospital Compare and the relevance of publicly reported data.

For Exercise 15.3, students discuss the Hospital Consumer Assessment of Healthcare Providers and Systems (HCAHPS). Instructors should guide students to explore the validity and reliability of HCAHPS as well as the challenges of using the tool.

For Exercise 15.4, students focus on how standardization and reliability have been achieved within the patient experience in a highly reliable organization. Students must search the literature for examples of standardized tools and patient involvement. Instructors should facilitate student discussion to link patient experience, patient involvement, and high reliability principles. The key for instructors is to look for examples of deference to expertise (involving patients) and then standardize practices for consistency.

These exercises can be accomplished in a discussion occurring in the physical classroom, in an online synchronous classroom, or in an instructor-prompted course-platform-based discussion board. These exercises could also be a graded paper.

STUDENT EVALUATION

Instructors should evaluate the following:

15.1 Was the student able to describe how patient experience is measured and improved within their practice environment?

15.2 Did the student compare the patient experience scores of three hospitals?

15.3 Was the student able to articulate a good understanding of the importance, measurement, and improvement efforts for patient experience?

15.4 Was the student able to find effective patient experience interventions and correlate their effectiveness with high reliability principles?

CHAPTER 16

PEDIATRIC PATIENT SAFETY: UTILIZING SAFETY COACHING AS A STRATEGY TOWARD ZERO HARM

In this chapter, students will learn about the difficulty of sustaining successful culture change. Students will also learn that taking culture change to the front line through peer safety coaches is an effective intervention to reinforce and sustain zero harm culture.

Chapter objective: Describe implementation of a safety coach program that improved and created a platform for sustainability of HRO principles within a pediatric environment.

Learning Activity 16.1 Examine the Role of Safety Coaches as a Vehicle for Successful Change Management and Sustainability of HRO Principles

Learning activity objectives:

16.1 Describe factors that influence change and challenges to change initiatives. (*applying*)

16.2 Describe the role of the patient safety coach and why it is needed for high reliability and sustained culture change. (*remembering*)

16.3 Examine challenges with peer coaching and suggest solutions. (*applying*)

Prior to completion of the learning activity, the student should do the following:

- Read Chapter 16.
- Read Caporale-Berkowitz, N., & Friedman, S. D. (2018). How peer coaching can make work less lonely. *Harvard Business Review*. Retrieved from https://hbr.org/2018/10/how-peer-coaching-can-make-work-less-lonely
- Watch the video *Peer to Peer Coaching:* https://www.ahrq.gov/hai/cusp/videos/07d-peer-2-peer-coach/index.html
- Read Kotter, J. (1995). Leading change: Why transformation efforts fail. *Harvard Business Review*, March–April 1995. Retrieved from https://oupub.etsu.edu/125/newbudgetprocess/documents/leading_change_why_transformation_efforts_fail.pdf

Instructions for learning activity exercises:

16.1 Describe a recent initiative that succeeded or failed within your organization. Correlate the success or failure to characteristics within a change model.

What was the initiative?

Who led the initiative?

How was the initiative received at the front line?

What tactics were used to spread the initiative and sustain the progress? Was a change model used? Which one?

Did the tactics succeed? Why?

Review the Kotter (1995) article. What failure factors from the article were evident in a failure or mitigated in a success? What could have been done differently?

16.2 Examine the role of the safety coach and how safety coaches can create sustainability of a zero-harm initiative.

Find and discuss a definition of a healthcare patient safety coach.

What are the challenges with giving feedback to peers?

Which is more successful: positive or negative feedback?

What kind of training do safety coaches need?

How can the role be supported to sustain gains in patient safety and quality?

Describe the benefits to a safety coach program within an organization to achieve a culture change to high reliability. How is coaching from a peer different from coaching from a supervisor?

16.3 Practice safety coaching using an example from the table or your own example to reinforce a desired safety behavior.

	What Did You Observe?	**What Is the Expectation?**	**How Would You Coach?**
Hand hygiene: Staff member does not practice hand hygiene.	Example: Staff member does not practice hand hygiene when entering a room.	Hand hygiene is expected when entering a room.	"Observations on your hand hygiene are always excellent, and I know that it is important to you. I noticed that this morning you didn't perform hand hygiene prior to going into Mr. Jones's room. Was there something else going on that was a distraction?"
Prevention of falls: Staff member leaves the room and does not set the bed alarm.	Example: You are doing rounds and find a bed alarm not set. The family member says that the nurse got called out of the room emergently after getting the patient back in bed.	Bed alarm is set.	"I was rounding and noticed that the bed alarm on Mr. Jones was not set. You always ensure that your high-risk fall patients are safe. I know you got called out of the room quickly. Is there a way that we could design a process to ensure that when someone gets called out of a high-risk room, another staff member can go in and check to see if all safety measures are in place?"
Protecting confidentiality: You hear staff members talking about a patient in the elevator.			
Effective communication: You witness a peer using a repeat-back to clarify an order.			
Asking questions: You hear a peer clarifying an unclear order.			

LEARNING ACTIVITY IMPLEMENTATION

Students will benefit most from these learning activities when they do them individually rather than in a group.

For Exercise 16.1, students should discuss principles of successful changes models. Instructors should guide students to apply a change model to an organization initiative and analyze the outcome of the initiative within the context of the selected change model.

For Exercise 16.2, students focus on the role of the safety coach. Students should articulate the value of a safety coach program for sustainability. Instructors should guide students to include practical challenges when providing peer-to-peer feedback.

For Exercise 16.3, students practice peer coaching through examples. Instructors should guide students to reflect on how it feels to practice peer coaching. This is an independent activity. However, student examples can be practiced in small groups.

These exercises can be accomplished in a discussion occurring in the physical classroom, in an online synchronous classroom, or in an instructor-prompted course-platform-based discussion board. Small groups may be conducive to practicing peer coaching.

STUDENT EVALUATION

Instructors should evaluate the following:

16.1 Was the student able to understand and explain how successful change occurs and relate these factors to a previous initiative?

16.2 Was the student able to articulate how a safety coach program can embed culture change and sustain an HRO initiative?

16.3 Was the student able to discuss methods to provide peer-to-peer safety coaching and address challenges?

PART 6

HRO CONCEPTS AND APPLICATION TO PRACTICE: RESILIENCE

Course objective: Recommend quality and safety activities based on high reliability principles. (*evaluating*)

CHAPTER 17

RESILIENCE: A PATH TO HRO

In this chapter, students will learn about the concept of resilience. Students will also learn resilience building strategies in the context of high reliability.

Chapter objective: Examine personal and organizational resilience-building strategies in the context of high reliability organizations (HROs).

Learning Activity 17.1: Resilience: Comparing Personal and Organizational Resilience in the Context of High Reliability

Learning activity objectives:

17.1 Describe the concept of resilience. (*understanding*)

17.2 Compare personal and organizational resilience-building strategies in the context of high reliability. (*analyzing*)

Prior to completion of the learning activity, the student should do the following:

- Read Chapter 17.
- Review Duke University Health System. (n.d.). Duke Center for Healthcare Safety and Quality. Retrieved from https://www.hsq.dukehealth.org/

Instructions for learning activity exercises:

17.1 Describe the concept of resilience and identify three personal resilience strategies. Complete one resilience tool offered at https://www.hsq.dukehealth.org/tools/

Describe the concept of resilience.
Describe the resilience tool offered by Duke Center for Healthcare Safety and Quality that you completed.
What did you learn about your personal resiliency?
Based on the outcome of the resilience tool, name three personal resilience strategies. Be prepared to discuss. 1. 2. 3.

17.2 Explain three resilience-building strategies at your organization in the context of high reliability.

Organization Resilience-Building Strategy	High Reliability Context
Team training programs	TeamSTEPPS training: Identifies barriers to effective teamwork. Training provides tools and strategies to enhance functioning of teams. High-functioning teams contribute to organizational resilience by maintaining a high level of performance despite environmental pressures.

LEARNING ACTIVITY IMPLEMENTATION

Students will benefit most from these learning activities when they do them individually rather than in a group.

For Exercise 17.1, students describe the concept of resilience and identify personal resilience strategies. Students must complete one resilience tool offered by Duke Center for Healthcare Safety and Quality and include how the resilience tool applies to their personal resilience strategies.

For Exercise 17.2, students identify and explain resilience strategies employed in their organization. Students must differentiate organization resilience strategies from personal resilience strategies described in Learning Activity 17.1. In the discussion, students should link organization resilience strategies to high reliability.

These exercises can be accomplished in a discussion occurring in the physical classroom, in an online synchronous classroom, or in an instructor-prompted course-platform-based discussion board. Also, instructors may consider these exercises as a graded paper or student presentation to the class.

STUDENT EVALUATION

Instructors should evaluate the following:

17.1 Was the student able to describe the concept of resilience? Was the student able to identify personal resilience strategies following completion of one resilience tool offered online by Duke Center for Healthcare Safety and Quality?

17.2 Was the student able to link organization resilience-building strategies and high reliability principles?

CHAPTER 18

DESIGNING RESILIENCE INTO THE WORK ENVIRONMENT

In this chapter, students will learn about a social-ecological perspective of resilience. Students will also learn to relate this perspective to high reliability, design a resilient work environment, and associate individual and work environment resilience with clinician well-being.

Chapter objective: Discover a social-ecological perspective of resilience to support clinician well-being.

Learning Activity 18.1: Apply a Social-Ecological Perspective of Resilience to Support Clinician Well-Being in the Work Environment

Learning activity objectives:

18.1 Describe resilience and how it relates to high reliability. (*understanding*)

18.2 Discuss opportunities for designing a resilient work environment. (*understanding*)

18.3 Associate individual and work environment resilience with clinician well-being. (*understanding*)

Prior to completion of the learning activity, the student should do the following:

- Read Chapter 18.
- Read National Academies of Sciences, Engineering, and Medicine. (2019). *Taking action against clinician burnout: A systems approach to professional well-being.* Washington, DC: The National Academies Press. https://doi.org/10.17226/25521

Instructions for learning activity exercises:

18.1 Describe resilience in your organization in the context of high reliability.

Resilience in my organization is:

18.2 Discuss three strategies to design a more resilient work environment in your organization. Include tactics to facilitate clinician well-being.

Work Environment Resilience Strategy	Tactics to Facilitate Clinician Well-Being
Leadership	Listens
	Practices stewardship to others
	Shows empathy
Culture	Respect
	Professionalism
Community	Providing and receiving social support
	Healing at the center of healthcare

18.3 Give three examples of how individual and work environment resilience affect clinician well-being within a social-ecological perspective of resilience.

Social-Ecological Perspective	Individual Resilience	Workplace Environment Resilience	Clinician Well-Being Influence
Individual	Maintaining a healthy diet	Healthy foods offered in cafeteria at reasonable price	Staying healthy
Team resilience	Good stress management routines	Being alert to overload	Work-life balance
Organization resilience	Good stress management	Ability of clinical unit to accept a sudden influx of patients	Maintain safety and quality
Society external environment	Professional factors	Organization shares a common leadership approach to professional policy	Mitigate burnout

LEARNING ACTIVITY IMPLEMENTATION

Students will benefit most from these learning activities when they do them individually rather than in a group.

For Exercise 18.1, students describe resilience in the context of high reliability in their organization. Students must link the concept of resilience and high reliability.

For Exercise 18.2, students discuss three strategies that could be employed at their organization to design a more resilient work environment. Exercise 18.2 builds on the description of resilience from Learning Activity 18.1. Instructors should coach discussion to include association of work environment resilience strategies and tactics that could facilitate clinician well-being.

For Exercise 18.3, students provide examples of individual and work environment resilience and discuss how their examples influence clinician well-being. Instructors should facilitate discussion framed in the social-ecological perspective explained in the chapter narrative and depicted in Figure 18.1 of the main book.

These exercises can be accomplished in a discussion occurring in the physical classroom, in an online synchronous classroom, or in an instructor-prompted course-platform-based discussion board. Also, instructors may consider these exercises as a graded paper or student presentation to the class.

STUDENT EVALUATION

Instructors should evaluate the following:

18.1 Was the student able to describe resilience in the context of high reliability?

18.2 Was the student able to discuss and associate work environment resiliency strategies with tactics that facilitate clinician well-being?

18.3 Was the student able to provide examples of how individual and work environment resilience affect well-being within the social-ecological framework?

CHAPTER 19

BUILDING HIGH RELIABILITY THROUGH SIMULATION

In this chapter, students will learn about healthcare simulation and blend simulation with the concepts of high reliability to create a view of simulation that improves the safety of high-risk processes. Students will also learn about the benefits of employing simulation as an advanced quality improvement and patient safety tool.

Chapter objective: Describe the emergence of simulation in schools, hospitals, and healthcare organizations as an advanced quality improvement and patient safety tool.

Learning Activity 19.1: Explore Opportunities to Use Simulation to Improve Safety and Reliability of Risk-Prone Processes

Learning activity objectives:

19.1 Compare and contrast traditional simulation and simulation designed for high reliability. (*analyzing*)

19.2 Apply simulation to a high-risk process
to improve the safety of the process. (*applying*)

Prior to completion of the learning activity, the student should do the following:

- Read Chapter 19.

- Find one peer-reviewed research article that applies simulation to a clinical safety or quality problem.

- Explore the website Clinical Simulation in Nursing at https://www.nursingsimulation.org/ for simulation articles and resources.

Instructions for learning activity exercises:

19.1 Describe the difference between traditional simulation such as experienced for learning competencies and simulation to improve safety of a high-risk process.

List some high-risk processes from your experience that might benefit from a simulation exercise.

How have these processes been practiced or simulated in your organization?

Were the practice sessions realistic?

Did the practice identify areas for improvement in teamwork, communication, or critical thinking?

Did the practice identify potential failures that might occur in the process?

Did participants in the practice session feel psychologically safe to speak up?

Did debriefing occur after the practice session?

Pick one of the high-risk processes that you currently practice or drill in your facility. Redesign the practice or drill to create a simulation that identifies safety issues within the process and increases the safety of the process.

Describe how simulation could be combined with an FMEA to identify failure modes.

19.2 Present your research article:

What was the practice problem that the simulation addressed?

Describe the method used for simulation.

What were the objectives and outcomes of the simulation?

Identify a high reliability principle that the simulation addressed or could have addressed.

LEARNING ACTIVITY IMPLEMENTATION

Students will benefit most from these learning activities when they do them individually rather than in a group.

For Exercise 19.1, students explore the world of simulation and how it can be used to effectively increase safety and improve quality. Instructors guide students to compare traditional simulation that simply reflects practice and simulation designed to identify failures and encourage teamwork and resilience.

For Exercise 19.2, students present peer-reviewed research articles that apply simulation to a clinical safety or quality problem. Instructors should guide the discussion to more fully explore simulation as a specialty practice.

These exercises can be accomplished in a discussion occurring in the physical classroom, in an online synchronous classroom, or in an instructor-prompted course-platform-based discussion board. Also, instructors may consider these exercises as a graded paper or a student presentation to the class.

STUDENT EVALUATION

Instructors should evaluate the following:

19.1 Was the student able to describe simulation for competency and simulation for high reliability?

19.2 Was the student able to identify opportunities for improved simulation of a high-risk process within the practice?

CHAPTER 20

BUILDING RESILIENCE THROUGH TEAM TRAINING: RAPID RESPONSE AND IN-HOSPITAL CARDIAC ARREST EVENTS

In this chapter, students will assess and evaluate the role resilience plays through team training events. Students will practice with an in-depth example of a healthcare emergency where multiple team members manage the emergency.

Chapter objective: Explain and evaluate how the high reliability principle of resilience improves team response to a cardiac event.

Learning Activity 20.1: Evaluate Rapid Response and In-Hospital Cardiac Arrest Event Team Performance

Learning activity objectives:

20.1   Evaluate rapid response and in-hospital cardiac arrest event team performance. (*evaluating*)

20.2   Explain team resilience gap analysis. (*analyzing*)

Prior to completion of the learning activity, the student should do the following:

- Read Chapter 20.
- Read Spitzer, C. R., Evans, K., Buehler, J., Ali, N. A., & Besecker, B. Y. (2019). Code blue pit crew model: A novel approach to in-hospital cardiac arrest resuscitation. *Resuscitation*, *143*, pp. 158–164.

Instructions for learning activity exercises:

20.1   Prepare an in-hospital cardiac arrest event team debrief using the Post Code Pause structured format. Include team resilience gap analysis in your discussion.

Date:_____ Age of Patient_____ Type of Alert:_____

Names of all staff members involved in post resuscitation pause

_____   _____

_____   _____   _____

**After the Event, everyone pauses for 10 seconds of silence to either remember the life of the person or celebrate the success of the Code Blue

What did the team do well?

What intervention(s) do you wish had or had not been offered?

How is your satisfaction with the equipment and medications available?

Where can we grow and improve?

How did we support the family (if they are present)?

How are you doing after the code?

What do you need to be able to be successful for returning to work right now?

Additional comments or concerns:

20.2 Prepare a rapid response event team debrief using the "What's Right?" structured format. Include team resilience gap analysis in your discussion.

The team leader will ask:

- Identify two things that went well in this RRT.
- Identify anything we can do to improve our RRT.

Each team member will be encouraged to share thoughts and new ideas.

RESILIENCE QUALITIES TO CONSIDER DURING GAP ANALYSIS

Indicator	Present	Absent	Follow-Up	Outcome Date
Are red-flag events or near misses reported?				
Is reporting of red-flag events rewarded?				
Is reporting of red-flag events punished?				
Have suggestions for workflow come from the workforce level?				
Do team meetings allow time for open discussion of everyday processes?				
Is the workflow regularly observed and evaluated by others?				
Does this process allow variation, or is variation open to safety issues?				
Have there been action-based mock drills?				
Are preprocess briefings used regularly?				
Are postevent debriefings used regularly?				
Is crew resource management training used with supervisors, and are the results monitored by leadership?				
Are stressful events (with or without outcome errors) reviewed?				
Are predictable workforce stressors identified and mitigated?				
After error mitigation, is the goal to return to steady state?				
Are the values of safety supported on every level of the workforce?				
Is data about safety, productivity, or processes well known and understood at all levels of the workforce?				

LEARNING ACTIVITY IMPLEMENTATION

Students will benefit most from these learning activities when they do them in a group rather than individually.

For Exercise 20.1, the instructor should provide a video simulation of a mock in-hospital cardiac arrest event for students to view. Divide or assign students to groups to view the video simulation, and then have each group of students prepare a debrief using the Post Code Pause structured format. Students should be prepared to present their observations and discuss opportunities to improve in-hospital cardiac arrest team performance, including team resilience gap analysis.

For Exercise 20.1, the instructor should provide a video simulation of a rapid response event for students to view. Divide or assign students to groups to view the video simulation, and then have each group of students prepare a debrief using the debriefing tool "What's Right?" structured format. Students should be prepared to present their observations and discuss opportunities to help the simulation team define their strengths and areas for growth, including team resilience gap analysis.

These exercises can be accomplished in a discussion occurring in the physical classroom, in an online synchronous classroom, or in an instructor-prompted course-platform-based discussion board.

STUDENT EVALUATION

Instructors should evaluate the following:

20.1 Were students able to prepare an in-hospital cardiac arrest event team debrief using the Post Code Pause structured format reflective of the event in the simulation video? Did they include resilience strategies in the discussion?

20.2 Were students able to prepare a rapid response event team debrief using the "What's Right?" structured format reflective of the event in the simulation video? Did they include resilience strategies in the discussion?

CHAPTER 21

SUSTAINING THE CULTURE OF SAFETY: STRATEGIES TO MAINTAIN THE GAINS

In this chapter, students will learn how resilient organizations can sustain a culture of safety by creating an organizational culture of personal and professional accountability.

Chapter objective: Explore a framework for change with strategies to sustain and maintain the gains within a culture of safety.

Learning Activity 21.1: Sustaining a Culture of Safety in a Resilient Organization

Learning activity objectives:

21.1 Discuss organizational vulnerabilities, related performance, and adherence to regulations and policies across the care continuum as a rationale for sustaining a culture of safety. (*understanding*)

21.2 Apply a framework for change to sustain and maintain a culture of safety. (*applying*)

21.3 Explain strategies to maintain the gains within a culture of safety in a resilient organization. (*analyzing*)

Prior to completion of the learning activity, the student should do the following:

- Read Chapter 21.
- Read Black, J. S. (2014). *It starts with one: Changing individuals changes organizations* (3rd ed.). Upper Saddle River, NJ: Pearson Education, Inc.

Instructions for learning activity exercises:

21.1 Discuss steps in developing culture change to support individual professional accountability and healthcare system performance.

21.2 Apply an evidence-based change model of your choice to a problem at your organization. Include barriers to change and mitigation strategies.

Change Model	Barriers to Change	Barrier Mitigation Strategies
Failure to see → What do we see?	Past successful mental maps "This is the way we do it here"	Clinical audit and feedback Peer review
Failure to move → How do we move?	New "right" thing not clearly identified Fear of appearing incompetent	Clear target identified Tools to help navigate to clear target—process improvement cycles
Failure to finish → How do we finish?	Fatigue—not going far enough or fast enough for change to succeed Majority do not adopt change	Champions to reinforce and encourage Majority adopt change

21.3 Name three strategies you could use after an evidence-based change to maintain and sustain gains in a culture of safety.

Strategy	Tactics
Leadership	Formal training
	Safety is strategic plan priority
	Active listening
Infrastructure and resource investment	Human factors engineer
	Internal governance and committee structure
Data analysis and feedback	Serious reportable events
	View multiple sources of data

LEARNING ACTIVITY IMPLEMENTATION

Students will benefit most from these learning activities when they do them in a group of four or five students.

For Exercise 21.1, students discuss the steps for developing culture change that support individual professional accountability and healthcare system performance. Students should include organizational vulnerabilities, related performance, and adherence to regulations and policies across the care continuum as a rationale for sustaining a culture of safety in their discussion.

For Exercise 21.2, students apply an evidence-based change model to a problem at their organization. The evidence-based change model for the learning activity is the student's choice. However, the model presented in Chapter 21 of the textbook is adequate for this activity. Instructors should guide students to include barriers to change and barrier mitigation strategies in EBP model application.

For Exercise 21.3, students name three strategies to maintain and sustain a culture of safety. The students should link strategies to maintain and sustain a culture of safety and organizational resilience in their discussion.

These exercises can be accomplished in a discussion occurring in the physical classroom, in an online synchronous classroom, or in an instructor-prompted course-platform-based discussion board. Also, instructors may consider these exercises as a student presentation to the class.

STUDENT EVALUATION

Instructors should evaluate the following:

21.1 Was the student able to discuss the steps to develop culture change? Did the student link individual professional accountability and health system performance to the steps of culture change?

21.2 Was the student able to select and apply an evidence-based change model to a problem at the organization? Did the student include barriers to change and mitigation strategies in the discussion?

21.3 Was the student able to name three strategies to sustain and maintain the gains following an evidence-based change?

PART 7

ASSIMILATION INTO PRACTICE ACROSS THE CONTINUUM

Course objective: Integrate high reliability principles into healthcare practice. (*creating*)

CHAPTER 22

APPLICATION OF HRO STRATEGIES TO IMPROVE PAIN MANAGEMENT AND OPIOID SAFETY: THE CNS ROLE

In this chapter, students will learn about how an advanced practice registered nurse can lead application of high reliability strategies to improve patient safety.

Chapter objective: Analyze the role of the advanced practice nurse in high reliability organizations.

Learning Activity 22.1: Examine Clinical Nurse Specialist Leadership of Clinical Improvement Teams in High Reliability Organizations

Learning activity objectives:

22.1 Discuss the value of the advanced practice registered nurse (APRN) in a high reliability organization. (*understanding*)

22.2 Explain the leadership role of the clinical nurse specialist in quality improvement. (*understanding*)

Prior to completion of the learning activity, the student should do the following:

- Read Chapter 22.
- Read Finkelman, A. (2013). The clinical nurse specialist: Leadership in quality improvement. *Clinical Nurse Specialist*, 27(1), pp. 31–35.

Instructions for learning activity exercises:

22.1 Identify a clinical quality improvement team led by an APRN at your organization and attend one meeting.

Clinical quality improvement team meeting:

Date:

Time:

APRN leader:

APRN leader role: (CNS, NP, CNM, CRNA)

22.2 Discuss how the APRN role uniquely leads and contributes to the quality improvement team. Include sources of evidence and linkage to high reliability principles.

APRN Contribution to QI Team	APRN Core Competencies	Link to High Reliability
CNS: Leader	Direct Patient Care: Evaluates impact of nursing interventions on patients' aggregate outcomes using a scientific approach.	Appreciate that small things going wrong are early warning signs.
	Source of evidence: NACNS CNS Core Competencies	

LEARNING ACTIVITY IMPLEMENTATION

Students will benefit most from these learning activities when they do them individually rather than in a group.

For Exercise 22.1, students identify a quality improvement team led by an APRN at their organization. The APRN leader could be a clinical nurse specialist, nurse practitioner, nurse midwife, or nurse anesthetist. The student should attend one meeting to observe APRN leadership of the group.

For Exercise 22.2, students build on Learning Activity 22.1 through evidence-based discussion of the APRN role and contribution to quality improvement activities. Students should be able to present evidence of core competencies for the specific APRN role and how these core competencies link to high reliability principles. The Consensus Model for APRN Regulation may be used as a source of evidence on licensure, accreditation, certification, and education for APRNs.

These exercises can be accomplished in a discussion occurring in the physical classroom, in an online synchronous classroom, or in an instructor-prompted course-platform-based discussion board. Also, instructors may consider these exercises as a graded paper or student presentation to the class.

STUDENT EVALUATION

Instructors should evaluate the following:

22.1 Was the student able to identify a quality improvement team led by an APRN at the organization? Was the student able to attend one meeting?

22.2 Was the student able to discuss the unique contributions of APRN leadership for the quality improvement team?

CHAPTER 23

AMBULATORY CARE: THE FRONTIER FOR HIGH RELIABILITY

In this chapter, students will learn about how high reliability principles can be used to address key quality and safety challenges in ambulatory care. Students will learn about the scope of ambulatory services as well as some of the unique complexities and challenges of this specialty.

Chapter objective: Discover how the principles of high reliability can mitigate quality and safety challenges in the ambulatory care setting.

Learning Activity 23.1: Integration of High Reliability Principles to Address Quality and Safety Challenges in Ambulatory Care

Learning activity objectives:

23.1 Discuss the scope of ambulatory services and the varied ambulatory settings. (*understanding*)

23.2 Explain complexities and challenges of ambulatory care. (*understanding*)

23.3 Articulate how each of the principles of high reliability can be used to mitigate quality and safety challenges in the ambulatory care space. (*applying*)

Prior to completion of the learning activity, the student should do the following:

- Read Chapter 23.
- Read Organisation for Economic Co-operation and Development. (2018). *The economics of patient safety in primary and ambulatory care.* Paris, France: OECD Publishing. Retrieved from https://www.oecd.org/health/health-systems/The-Economics-of-Patient-Safety-in-Primary-and-Ambulatory-Care-April2018.pdf

Instructions for learning activity exercises:

23.1 Choose an ambulatory care setting in your organization. Include the rationale for your choice.

23.2 Identify at least three complexities and challenges of the chosen ambulatory care setting.

23.3 Create a table integrating high reliability principles that can mitigate complexities and challenges of the chosen ambulatory care setting.

Ambulatory Care Setting: Ambulatory Infusion Center

Rationale: Outpatient administration of infusible and injectable pharmacological and biological agents. I work there.

Complexities	Unique Safety Challenges	High Reliability Solution
Diverse care team of interprofessional experts	Skill mix and delegation	Deference to expertise Clear role delineation Daily huddles
Communication gaps	Medication administration errors	Preoccupation with failure Systematic approach to reviewing errors
Care transition management	Care coordination	Sensitivity to operations Standardizing workflows and communication

LEARNING ACTIVITY IMPLEMENTATION

Students will benefit most from these learning activities when they do them individually rather than in a group.

For Exercise 23.1, students select an ambulatory care setting in their organization. Students must include a rationale for their choice.

For Exercise 23.2, students identify complexities and challenges of the ambulatory care setting from Exercise 23.1. Instructors should facilitate discussion to include a variety of ambulatory care settings.

For Exercise 23.3, students are building on Exercise 23.1 and Exercise 23.2 by integrating high reliability principles to mitigate complexities and challenges unique to the selected ambulatory care setting. Students should be able to generate a table that links high reliability principles and strategies to mitigate complexities and challenges of the selected ambulatory care setting.

These exercises can be accomplished in a discussion occurring in the physical classroom, in an online synchronous classroom, or in an instructor-prompted course-platform-based discussion board. Also, instructors may consider these exercises as a graded paper or student presentation to the class.

STUDENT EVALUATION

Instructors should evaluate the following:

23.1 Was the student able to select an ambulatory care setting in the organization? Was rationale for choice of setting included?

23.2 Was the student able to identify a minimum of three complexities and challenges of the chosen ambulatory care setting?

23.3 Was the student able to create a table integrating high reliability principles that could mitigate complexities and challenges of the selected ambulatory care setting?

CHAPTER 24

APPLYING HIGH RELIABILITY PRINCIPLES ACROSS A LARGE HEALTHCARE SYSTEM TO REDUCE PATIENT FALLS

In this chapter, students will learn about how high reliability principles can be used in large multihospital systems to improve patient safety. Students will also learn how nurse-led initiatives, empowerment, and innovation advance the culture of patient safety.

Chapter objective: Explain how to leverage high reliability principles to improve patient safety.

Learning Activity 24.1: Apply High Reliability Tenets to Solve Health System Quality and Safety Challenges

Learning activity objectives:

24.1 Use high reliability organization characteristics to design a nursing practice change that improves a quality/safety measure. (*applying*)

24.2 Select a nurse-led quality/safety improvement opportunity where application of HR could make a positive impact. (*applying*)

24.3 Design a project plan using HR principles to improve the quality/safety opportunity. (*creating*)

Prior to completion of the learning activity, the student should do the following:

- Read Chapter 24.
- Identify a clinical quality improvement opportunity that could be affected by a nursing practice change.
- Read Oster, C. A., & Deakins, S. (2018). Practical application of high-reliability principles in healthcare to optimize quality and safety outcomes. *Journal of Nursing Administration*, *48*(1), pp. 50–55.

Instructions for learning activity exercises:

24.1 Identify a quality/safety improvement opportunity where nurses can make an impact through nursing practice changes through the use of HR principles.

24.2 Using knowledge of HR principles, explain which HR principles are relevant in solving the problem and why. Be prepared to discuss the link between nurse empowerment over practice and HR principles with your classmates.

Quality/Safety Improvement Need	Principle 1 Preoccupation With Failure	Principle 2 Reluctance to Simplify	Principle 3 Sensitivity to Operations	Principle 4 Commitment to Resilience	Principle 5 Deference to Expertise
Example: Reduce fall rates	When nurses constantly think about fall prevention, vigilance increases.	Reducing falls is a complex problem requiring intricate solutions.	Preventing patient falls is a team sport, requiring extensive interdependency between care providers and departments.	To ensure organizational commitment to reducing falls, a culture of continuous learning and support must be present.	Empowering clinical nurses with direct line of sight to patients leverages nursing expertise to solve a complex problem.

CHAPTER 24 APPLYING HIGH RELIABILITY PRINCIPLES ACROSS A LARGE HEALTHCARE SYSTEM TO REDUCE PATIENT FALLS

24.3 Design a nursing project plan using HR principles to improve the quality/safety opportunity. There are nine sections to complete for this activity.

Describe the quality/safety project.

Identify the project deliverables.

List the baseline measures related to the project.

Complete the project plan charter form.

List steps or approaches/ideas on how you, as the team leader, would ensure integration of the HR principles into the solution(s).

Describe any risks or threats to the project.

Briefly describe a communication plan for the project.

Briefly describe a training plan for the project.

Briefly describe how you would evaluate the project's success.

LEARNING ACTIVITY IMPLEMENTATION

Students will benefit the most from these learning activities when they do them in a group of four or five students.

For Exercise 24.1, students identify a quality/safety improvement opportunity where nurses can make an impact on nursing practice changes through the use of HR principles. The opportunity can be from their organization or from the literature.

For Exercise 24.2, students use high reliability organization characteristics to design a nursing practice change that improves a quality/safety measure by completing the table template. Students should include a discussion of the link between nurse empowerment over practice and high reliability principles.

For Exercise 24.3, students design a nursing project plan to address the quality/safety opportunity identified in Exercise 24.1. The nine-step project plan template is included in this guide.

These exercises can be accomplished in a discussion occurring in the physical classroom, in an online synchronous classroom, or in an instructor-prompted course-platform-based discussion board. Also, instructors may consider these exercises as a graded paper or a student presentation to the class.

STUDENT EVALUATION

Instructors should evaluate the following:

24.1 Was the student able to identify a quality/safety improvement opportunity where nurses can make an impact on nursing practice changes through the use of HR principles? Was the student able to document how nursing knowledge and expertise connect with each of the HR principles?

24.2 Did the student select a nurse-led quality/safety improvement opportunity where application of HR could make a positive impact?

24.3 Did the student design a project plan using HR principles to improve the quality/safety opportunity?

NINE-STEP PROJECT PLAN TEMPLATE

Potential Project Name/Title		Date	
Requested by		Charter Prepared by	

Background & Business Need: State the business problem/issue to solve or what opportunity exists to improve a business function. What is the current state? Narrative background with drivers for the project.

Project Scope Statement: Summarize the purpose and the intent of the project and describe what the customer (or you) envisions will be delivered.

Project Objectives/Deliverables: Outline the high-level objectives for the project. What will exist when the project is complete? Include the benefits of the project, including how the project will benefit the customers or stakeholders.

Boundaries: What will <u>not</u> be included in this project?

Assumptions: What assumptions were made when conceiving this project?

External Dependencies: Note any major external (to the project) dependencies the project must rely upon for success, such as specific technologies, third-party vendors, development partners, or other business relationships. Also identify any other related projects or initiatives.

Project Risks: List any known risks for the project that could impact the success of the project or should be considered when planning. Include risk of change management. Does the value of this project ultimately depend on people changing their work or behavior? Identify risks facing this project or organization if the people side of the project is poorly manned.

Key Stakeholders: List the key stakeholders for the project. Stakeholders are individuals, groups, or organizations that are actively involved in a project, are affected by its outcome, or can influence its outcome. Indicate their role or interest in the project. These stakeholders (or representatives) MAY be invited to participate in a project kickoff session but do not necessarily need to be on the project team. Whose day-to-day work will be impacted by raw processes (systems, tools, job roles, organization structure, etc.) as an outcome or deliverable of this project?

Stakeholder/Stakeholder Group	Role in Project or Impacted by This Project

Required Resources: Identify the known resources that management is willing to commit to the project at this time. Human resources includes key individuals, teams, organizations, subcontractors or vendors, and support functions. This is not the place for the detailed team staff roster for individual names. Identify critical skill sets that team members must have. Other resources could include funding, computers, other equipment, physical facilities such as buildings and rooms, hardware devices, software tools, and training. What level of change management involvement is expected for this project? (e.g., separate change management team, change management representation on the core team or individual team).

Requested Timeline/Milestones: Include end and start dates and key milestones.

CHAPTER

25

THE SYNTHESIS AMONG MAGNET RECOGNITION PROGRAM® MODEL COMPONENTS AND HIGH RELIABILITY ORGANIZATION PRINCIPLES

In this chapter, students will learn about how the Magnet® model component characteristics provide the foundation for synergistic relationships with high reliability organization (HRO) principles. Student will also learn about the synergy of Magnet components and high reliability principles.

Chapter objective: Discover how high reliability principles can be related to the components of the Magnet model.

Learning Activity 25.1: Explain the Synergistic Relationship Between the Magnet Model Components and the Principles of High Reliability

Learning activity objectives:

25.1 Describe the Magnet Recognition Program® components. (*understanding*)

25.2 Discuss the synergy of high reliability principles with Magnet Recognition Program components. (*understanding*)

Prior to completion of the learning activity, the student should do the following:

- Read Chapter 25.
- Read American Nurses Credentialing Center. (n.d.). ANCC Magnet Recognition Program®. Retrieved from https://www.nursingworld.org/organizational-programs/magnet/

Instructions for learning activity exercises:

25.1 Discuss the five components and component characteristics of the Magnet model.

Magnet Component	Description
Exemplary professional practice	Understanding of the role of nursing; autonomous practice based on competence; application of nursing role with patients, families, communities, and interprofessional teams; nurse partnerships to deliver patient-/person-centered care

25.2 Describe the synergy of high reliability principles and Magnet Recognition Program components and include examples of synergy.

Magnet Recognition Component/ Description	Example of Magnet Component From Organization	High Reliability Principle	Description of Synergy
Transformational leadership	Vision of elimination of patient harm	Preoccupation with failure	For the preoccupation with failure to work, there needs to be a high level of trust and communication within the organization. Leadership must take time to provide the "why" and encourage two-way feedback among management and staff, and it needs to be viewed as constructive. Leaders who take the time to answer why will produce a workforce with buy-in and one that is more flexible and responsive to change.

LEARNING ACTIVITY IMPLEMENTATION

Students will benefit most from these learning activities when they do them individually rather than in a group.

For Exercise 25.1, students should be able to name each of the five components of the Magnet model. Instructors should coach students to include description and component characteristics in their discussion.

For Exercise 25.2, students build on knowledge from Exercise 25.1. In this exercise, students describe the synergy of high reliability principles and Magnet Program Recognition components by providing examples from their organization. Instructors may need to coach students to link high reliability principles and Magnet Recognition Program components to examples in practice.

These exercises can be accomplished in a discussion occurring in the physical classroom, in an online synchronous classroom, or in an instructor-prompted course-platform-based discussion board.

STUDENT EVALUATION

Instructors should evaluate the following:

25.1 Was the student able to discuss the components of the Magnet model? Was the student able to discuss the characteristics of each component of the model?

25.2 Was the student able to provide practice examples describing the synergy of high reliability principles and Magnet Recognition Program components?

CHAPTER 26

ACHIEVING HRO: THE ROLE OF THE BEDSIDE SCIENTIST IN RESEARCH

In this chapter, students will learn about the culture of inquiry in a high reliability organization and the role of the bedside scientist in research. Students will also learn about barriers to research, overcoming barriers, and creating research infrastructure supporting the clinical/bedside nurse in the conduct of research in a highly reliable organization.

Chapter objective: Explain a culture of inquiry in a high reliability organization.

Learning Activity 26.1: Discover the Role of the Bedside Scientist in a High Reliability Organization

Learning activity objectives:

26.1 Describe the role of the bedside scientist in a high reliability organization. (*understanding*)

26.2 Discuss research barriers and strategies to overcome the barriers. (*understanding*)

Prior to completion of the learning activity, the student should do the following:

- Read Chapter 26.
- Read Ghaferi, A., Myers, C., Sutcliffe, K., & Pronovost, P. (2016). The next wave of hospital innovation to make patients safer. *Harvard Business Review*. Retrieved from https://hbr.org/2016/08/the-next-wave-of-hospital-innovation-to-make-patients-safer
- Read Hain, D. J., & Kear, T. M. (2015). Using evidence-based practice to move beyond doing things the way we have always done them. *Nephrology Nursing Journal, 42*(1), pp. 11–21.

Instructions for learning activity exercises:

26.1 Identify an opportunity for improvement or innovation at your organization, and conduct a brief literature review on the topic. Include three or four sources of peer-reviewed evidence.

Opportunity for improvement or innovation at your organization:

Source (author, title, year)	Purpose of Study	Method (including setting and sample)	Key Findings and Implications	Limitations of Study

26.2 Describe how a bedside scientist would advance the opportunity for improvement or innovation in a highly reliable organization.

Describe the role of the bedside scientist to advance the improvement or innovation idea:

Frontline bedside scientist:

Advanced practice nurse bedside scientist:

Doctorally prepared bedside scientist:

> Attend a patient safety, evidence-based practice, quality improvement, or research meeting related to an improvement or innovation topic to gain insight into the role of the bedside scientist.
>
> Meeting title:
>
> Date:
>
> Time:
>
> Reflection: (what occurred during the meeting integrating high reliability concepts)

LEARNING ACTIVITY IMPLEMENTATION

Students will benefit most from these learning activities when they do them either individually or in a group.

For Exercise 26.1, students should identify an opportunity for improvement or innovation at their organization. Students should conduct a brief literature review on the topic. Instructors should guide students to include three or four peer-reviewed sources of evidence on the improvement or innovation topic.

For Exercise 26.2, students build on Exercise 26.1. In this exercise students describe the role of the bedside scientist to advance the improvement or innovation idea. Description of the bedside scientist should mention frontline staff, advanced practice nurses, and doctorally prepared nurses. Instructors should guide students to link high reliability to a culture of inquiry. Students could attend a patient safety, evidence-based practice, quality improvement, or research meeting related to their topic to get insight into the role of the bedside scientist. Ask students to provide a reflection on what occurred during the meeting and what they thought about it in the context of high reliability.

These exercises can be accomplished in a discussion in the physical classroom, in an online synchronous classroom, or in an instructor-prompted course-platform-based discussion board. Instructors may consider these exercises as a presentation to the class.

STUDENT EVALUATION

Instructors should evaluate the following:

26.1 Was the student able to identify an opportunity for improvement or innovation at the organization? Was the student able to locate three or four peer-reviewed sources of evidence from the literature on the opportunity for improvement or innovation?

26.2 Was the student able to describe how the bedside scientist would advance the improvement or innovation idea? Was the student able to link high reliability to a culture of inquiry?

PART 8

TRANSLATION INTO PRACTICE

Course objective: Integrate high reliability principles into healthcare practice. (*creating*)

SUMMATIVE ASSESSMENT: TRANSLATION INTO PRACTICE

In Part 8, Chapters 27 to 32, students will learn about how staff at the front line of care identified problems in their specialty area and created an improvement project employing high reliability principles. Students will also learn how an evidence-based practice project is implemented to incorporate high reliability principles, evidence-based practice, and change management.

Section objective: Examine how high reliability principles are translated into practice.

Summative Learning Activity 27.1: Translate Evidence-Based Practice, Change Management, and High Reliability Principles to Practice

Summative learning activity objectives:

27.1 Identify an evidence-based practice model and a change model. (*understanding*)

27.2 Identify characteristics of evidence-based practice process, change management, and high reliability principles in one of the provided examples. (*understanding*)

27.3 Apply characteristics of evidence-based practice process, change management, and high reliability principles to a student-selected clinical practice problem. (*applying*)

Prior to completion of the learning activity, the student should do the following:

- Read Chapters 27–32.

Instructions for summative learning activity exercises:

27.1 Identify an evidence-based practice model and a change management model. Choose one chapter from the assigned readings. Using selected EBP and change management models, identify steps of the EBP process and change management process described in the chapter. Answer the following questions to evaluate the translation-into-practice example:

　How did the project use data to identify the need for change or define the problem?

　How was literature used to explain the rationale for the intervention?

　Is the intervention based on a theory?

　How did the authors obtain buy-in from stakeholders?

　Was there any evidence of resistance to change?

　How was resistance to change addressed?

　How was data collected and analyzed?

　Was a tool used for data collection?

　Is there a plan for sustainability?

27.2 Identify characteristics and use of high reliability principles within the aforementioned translation-into-practice example.

27.3 Identify a problem from your own practice and integrate evidence-based practice steps, change management principles, and high reliability principles to create a sustainable practice change.

Create a basic proposal to describe your plan. Include the following:
- Background and significance of the problem
- Problem statement
- Objectives and aims of the project; intervention description
- Methodology
- Proposed intervention
- Setting and participants
- Proposed outcome measures and evaluation
- Data collection plan
- Data analysis plan

Include a description of a tool or method of high reliability and a description of a principle of change management.

SUMMATIVE LEARNING ACTIVITY IMPLEMENTATION

Students should complete the summative learning activity exercises individually.

For Summative Exercise 27.1, students select one of the clinical translations-into-practice examples in the textbook. The student should be able to identify EBP process steps along with change management processes. The EBP Worksheet in the appendices of this guide may be helpful for students completing this exercise.

For Summative Exercise 27.2, students identify characteristics and use of high reliability principles within the selected translation-into-practice example. The student should be able to trace how high reliability principles were translated into practice. High Reliability Organizations: A Quick Guide for Frontline Application, located in the appendices of this guide, may be helpful for students to use to complete this exercise.

For Summative Exercise 27.3, each student prepares a draft proposal for a sustainable practice change. The proposal is comprehensive in nature. Instructors should guide students to translate high reliability principles discussed throughout the course into clinical practice. Students should integrate evidence-based practice steps, change management principles, and high reliability principles to create a sustainable practice change.

These exercises can be accomplished in a discussion in the physical classroom, in an online synchronous classroom, or in an instructor-prompted course-platform-based discussion board. Instructors may consider summative Exercises 27.1 and 27.2 as a presentation to the class. Summative Exercise 27.3 is intended as a graded paper with sources, in lieu of a final exam.

STUDENT EVALUATION

Instructors should evaluate the following:

27.1 Was the student able to identify steps of the EBP process and change management process in a translation-into-practice example?

27.2 Was the student able to identify characteristics and use of high reliability principles in a translation-into-practice example?

27.3 Was the student able to translate evidence-based practice, change management, and high reliability principles to draft a proposal for a sustainable practice change?

SUPPLEMENTAL INSTRUCTOR RESOURCES AND READINGS

PART 1

CHAPTER 1

Hollnagel, E. (2014). *Safety I and safety II: The past and future of safety management*. Boca Raton, FL: CRC.

Veazie, S., Peterson, K., & Bourne, D. (2019). Evidence brief: Implementation of high reliability organization principles. Washington, DC: Evidence Synthesis Program, Health Services Research and Development Service, Office of Research and Development, Department of Veterans Affairs. VA ESP Project #09-199. Retrieved from https://www.hsrd.research.va.gov/publications/esp/reports.cfm

CHAPTER 2

Armstrong, G., & Sherwood, G. (2020). Patient safety. In J. F. Giddens (Ed.), *Concepts for nursing practice* (pp. 434–442). St. Louis, MO: Elsevier.

Barnsteiner, J. (2017). Safety. In G. Sherwood & J. Barnsteiner (Eds.), *Quality and safety in nursing: A competency approach to improving outcomes* (pp. 149–170). Hoboken, NJ: Wiley-Blackwell.

Sherwood, G. (2017). Driving forces for quality and safety: Changing mindsets to improve healthcare. In G. Sherwood & J. Barnsteiner (Eds.), *Quality and safety in nursing: A competency approach to improving outcomes* (pp. 3–21). Hoboken, NJ: Wiley-Blackwell.

CHAPTER 3

Al-Amin, M., Schiaffino, M. K., Park, S., & Harman, J. (2018). Sustained hospital performance on consumer assessment of healthcare providers and system survey measures. What are the determinants? *Foundation of the American College of Healthcare Executives*, *36*(1), pp. 15–28. doi:10.1097/JHM-D-16-00006

CHAPTER 4

Chassin, M. R., & Loeb, J. M. (2013). High-reliability health care: Getting there from here. *The Milbank Quarterly*, *91*(3), pp. 459–490.

Schein, E. H. (2017). *Organizational culture and leadership* (5th ed.). San Francisco, CA: Jossey-Bass.

CHAPTER 5

Ford, J. L. (2018). Revisiting high-reliability organizing: Obstacles to safety and resilience. *Corporate Communications: An International Journal*, *23*(2), pp. 197–211.

Weick, K. E., & Sutcliffe, K. M. (2015). *Managing the unexpected: Sustaining performance in a complex world* (3rd ed.). Hoboken, NJ: John Wiley & Sons, Inc.

PART 2

CHAPTER 6

Centers for Medicare & Medicaid Services. (n.d). *Guidance for performing failure mode and effects analysis with performance improvement projects*. Retrieved from https://www.cms.gov/Medicare/Provider-Enrollment-and-Certification/QAPI/Downloads/GuidanceForFMEA.pdf

CHAPTER 7

The Joint Commission. (2018). *Developing a reporting culture: Learning from close calls and hazardous conditions*. Retrieved from https://www.jointcommission.org/-/media/tjc/documents/resources/patient-safety-topics/sentinel-event/sea_60_reporting_culture_final.pdf?db=web&hash=5AB072026CAAF4711FCDC343701B0159

PART 3

CHAPTER 8

Dekker, S. (2011). *Patient safety: A human factors approach*. Boca Raton, FL: CRC Press.

Marriott, R. D. (2018). Process mapping–The foundation for effective quality improvement. *Current Problems in Pediatric and Adolescent Health Care*, *48*(7), pp. 177–181.

CHAPTER 9

National Patient Safety Foundation. (2015). *RCA²: Improving root cause analyses and actions to prevent harm.* Retrieved from http://www.ihi.org/resources/Pages/Tools/RCA2-Improving-Root-Cause-Analyses-and-Actions-to-Prevent-Harm.aspx

Reason, J. T. (1997). *Managing the risks of organizational accidents.* Farnham, UK: Ashgate Publishing Company.

CHAPTER 10

Marx, D. (2009). *Whack a mole: The price we pay for expecting perfection.* Plano, TX: By Your Side Studios.

Dekker, S. (2013). *Second victim: Error, guilt, trauma and resilience.* Boca Raton, FL: Chapman and Hall/CRC.

Dekker, S. (2016). *Just Culture: Restoring trust and accountability in your organization* (3rd ed.). Boca Raton, FL: CRC Press.

PART 4

CHAPTER 11

ECRI Institute. (2020). *Top ten health technology hazards.* Retrieved from https://www.ecri.org/landing-2020-top-ten-health-technology-hazards/

CHAPTER 12

Englebright, J. (2019). *Ideal nursing workflows to support the development of information technology solutions.* Virginia Henderson Global Nursing e-Repository. Retrieved from http://hdl.handle.net/10755/17235

CHAPTER 13

Goldenhar, L. M., Brady, P. W., Sutcliffe, K. M., & Muething, S. E. (2013). Huddling for high reliability and situation awareness. *BMJ Quality and Safety, 22*(11), pp. 899–906.

PART 5

CHAPTER 14

Rosen, M. A., DiazGranados, D., Dietz, A. S., Benishe, L. E., Pronovost, P. J., & Weaver, S. J. (2018). Teamwork in healthcare: Key discoveries enabling safer, high quality care. *American Psychologist; 73*(4), pp. 433–450.

CHAPTER 15

Dempsey, C. (2017). *The antidote to suffering: How compassionate connected care can improve safety, quality, and experience.* New York, NY: McGraw-Hill Education.

CHAPTER 16

Kotter, J. (1995, March–April). Leading change: Why transformation efforts fail. *Harvard Business Review.* Retrieved from https://oupub.etsu.edu/125/newbudgetprocess/documents/leading_change_why_transformation_efforts_fail.pdf

PART 6

CHAPTER 17

Obenrader, C., Broome, M. E., Yap, T. L., & Jamison, F. (2019). Changing team member perceptions by implementing TeamSTEPPS in an emergency department. *Journal of Emergency Nursing, 45*(1), pp. 31–37.

CHAPTER 18

National Academies of Sciences, Engineering, and Medicine (2019). *Taking action against clinician burnout: A systems approach to professional well-being*. Washington, DC: The National Academies Press. Retrieved from https://doi.org/10.17226/25521

CHAPTER 19

The Society for Simulation in Healthcare contains multiple resources. See https://www.ssih.org/.

CHAPTER 20

Williams, K-L., Rideout, J., Pritchett-Kelly, J., McDonald, M., Mullins-Richards, M., & Dubrowski, A. (2016). Mock code: A code blue scenario requested by and developed for registered nurses. *Cureus, 8*(12), p. e938.

CHAPTER 21

Black, J. S. (2014). *It starts with one: Changing individuals changes organizations* (3rd ed.). Upper Saddle River, NJ: Pearson Education, Inc.

Dekker, S. (2016). *Just Culture—Restoring trust and accountability in your organization* (3rd ed.). Boca Raton, FL: CRC Press.

PART 7

CHAPTER 22

American Association of Colleges of Nursing. (n.d.). APRN Consensus Model. Retrieved from https://www.aacnnursing.org/Education-Resources/APRN-Education/APRN-Consensus-Model

Finkelman, A. (2013). The clinical nurse specialist: Leadership in quality improvement. *Clinical Nurse Specialist, 27*(1), pp. 31–35.

CHAPTER 23

Gaguski, M. E., & Nguyen, H. T. (2016). An interdisciplinary approach to the development and implementation of electronic treatment orders in a medical oncology department. *Clinical Journal of Oncology Nursing, 20*(4), pp. 371–373.

CHAPTER 24

Adelman, J. (2019). High-reliability healthcare: Building safer systems through Just Culture and technology. *Journal of Healthcare Management, 64*(3), pp. 137–141.

CHAPTER 25

American Nurses Credentialing Center. (2018). *2019 Magnet® application manual*. Silver Spring, MD: Author.

CHAPTER 26

Houser, J., & Bokovoy, J. L. (2006). *Clinical research in practice: A guide for the bedside scientist*. Sudbury, MA: Jones & Bartlett Publishers.

Logsdon, M. C., Kleiner, C., Oster, C. A., Smith, C. D., Bergman-Evans, B., Kempnich, J. M.,…Meyers, J. (2017). Description of nurse scientists in a large health care system. *Nursing Administration Quarterly, 41*(3), pp. 266–274. doi:10.1097/NAQ.0000000000000237

PART 8

CHAPTERS 27–32

Cullen, L., Hanrahan, K., Farrington, M., DeBerg, J., Kleiber, C., & Tucker, S. (2018). *Evidence-based practice in action: Comprehensive strategies, tools, and tips from the University of Iowa Hospitals and Clinics*. Indianapolis, IN: Sigma Theta Tau International.

Houser, J., & Oman, K. (Eds.). (2011). *Evidence-based practice: An implementation guide for healthcare organizations*. Boston, MA: Jones and Bartlett.

Mazurek-Melnyk, B., & Fineholt-Overholt, E. (2019). *Evidence-based practice in nursing & healthcare: A guide to best practice* (4th ed.). Philadelphia, PA: Wolters Kluwer.

APPENDICES

Appendix A:
EBP Worksheet

Appendix B:
High Reliability Organizations:
A Quick Guide for Frontline Application

Appendix A: EBP Worksheet

Project Title		
Name (Stakeholders)	Unit	Title

Unit Manager's Name and Work

Problem Identified: What is a problem you see at your work? NDNQI, such as PI, Fall, CAUTI? What is your current number? How are you able to obtain that?

Patient Outcome: What is the patient outcome expected to improve? How are you going to measure?

Process Outcome: What is the process outcome to assess effectiveness of your project? How are you going to measure?

PICO Concepts for Developing a Purpose Statement

Patient Population

Clinical **P**roblem or Condition (include numbers to support, such as fall rate or CAUTI rate)

Interventions

What do you want to implement?

How do you want to implement?

Comparison

Anticipated **O**utcomes (Process Outcome and Patient Outcome)

Patient Outcome

Process Outcome

Next Steps

Your Work Plan/Next Steps

-
-
-

Appendix B: High Reliability Organizations: A Quick Guide for Frontline Application

Objectives for the user of this guide:

- Understand the concept of high reliability organizations (HROs) and their application to patient safety.
- Explain the five principles of HROs as described by Weick and Sutcliffe.
- Apply the principles to your work area by discussing key questions.
- Use a guide to identify a process in your work area that requires high reliability.
- Use a guide to analyze and improve the process by using high reliability techniques.

What Are High Reliability Organizations (HROs)?

High reliability organizations are those that are high-risk, dynamic, turbulent, and potentially hazardous, yet operate nearly error-free. Examples include aviation, nuclear engineering, defense operations, and acute care hospitals.

How do high reliability organizations stay error free?

- HROs recognize that small things that go wrong are often early warning signs of trouble. The warning signs are the "red flags" that provide insight into the health of the whole system.
- HROs value near misses as indicators of early trouble and are acted on to prevent future failure. Near misses are not seen as an indicator of system success.
- HROs are innovative and creative, and they value input from all corners of the organization.
- HROs recognize the value of preparing for the unexpected and the unknown. Failures rarely occur if they are expected.

The five principles of hROs follow:

- **Preoccupation with failure:** HROs are preoccupied with all failures, especially small ones. Small things that go wrong are often early warning signals of deepening trouble and give insight into the health of the whole system. But we have a tendency to ignore or overlook our failures (which suggest we are not competent) and focus on our successes (which suggest we are competent).
- **Reluctance to simplify:** HROs restrain their temptation to simplify through diverse checks and balances, adversarial reviews, and the cultivation of multiple perspectives.
- **Sensitivity to operations:** HROs make strong responses to weak signals (indications that something might be amiss). Everyone values organizing to maintain situational awareness.
- **Commitment to resilience:** HROs pay close attention to their capability to improvise and act—without knowing in advance what will happen.
- **Deference to expertise:** HROs shift decisions away from formal authority toward expertise and experience. Decision-making migrates to experts at all levels of the hierarchy during high tempo times.

HIGH RELIABILITY ORGANIZATION CHARACTERISTICS*

PREOCCUPATION WITH FAILURE

What is preoccupation with failure?

Preoccupation with failure is a determined mind-set to continually watch the system for subtle signs or weak signals of failure. An analogy is the prevention of forest fires: Look for and put out the spark before the fire. Systems with high reliability worry persistently that small errors are rooted in routine work and that unexpected events and limitations of foresight may intensify these errors.

Why is preoccupation with failure important to high reliability?

High reliability means that the expected outcome occurs every time. For example, the outcome of a pilot landing a passenger airplane safely is expected every time. Due to unexpected events and hidden failures, a plane landing successfully once does not mean that it will land successfully in the future. Adverse events in the hospital follow the same course. Adverse events occur in routine and previously successful procedures and processes due to events that were not anticipated and a buildup of hidden or weak failures.

Although success is desirable, it can breed overconfidence and cause blind spots. High reliability organizations do not ignore successful operations as resistant to failure. High reliability organizations take successful operations and continue to look for and correct unanticipated failures before they occur.

Why is preoccupation with failure challenging to healthcare organizations?

Hospitals need for consumers, staff, and payers to see high-quality care to remain financially viable. Bad news or signs of failure can be perceived as a sign of incompetence or lack of quality. However, adverse events to patients can be prevented when organizations consider "bad news" such as early identification of signs of failure as "good news" because it leads to correction of the problem prior to a total breakdown.

What are some hospital examples of preoccupation with failure?

- Calling the RRT for a subtle sign of clinical deterioration and moving the patient to the ICU prior to a resuscitation
- Reporting near misses and digging deeper to find out why they occur and how the problem could be corrected prior to reaching a patient
- Conducting Failure Mode Effects Analysis (FMEA) prior to and after implementation of new equipment or processes to determine latent or weak failures in the system

---

* Weick, K., & Sutcliffe, K. (2015). *Managing the unexpected: Sustained performance in a complex world* (3rd ed.). Hoboken, NJ: Jossey-Bass.

Is your unit/work area preoccupied with failure? Ask:

- Are we rewarded when we report mistakes, near misses? Is it easy to report a near miss?
- What near misses were reported here, and did we change anything because of the near miss? Why or why not?

RELUCTANCE TO SIMPLIFY

What is reluctance to simplify?

Failures seldom occur without early warning signs. Early warning signs of problems are easily missed when the focus is on quick solutions based on a narrow or predetermined viewpoint. More often, the solution is found within the full context or the details of a situation. Reluctance to simplify means that problems are solved by asking more questions from diverse viewpoints to paint a richer picture of the problem. Solutions are generated by refusing to categorize the problem until it is fully described.

Why is reluctance to simplify important to high reliability?

High reliability organizations work to become experts at handling unexpected events. Unexpected events come from diverse pathways. Diversity is needed to fully explore the range of these unexpected events. For example, if nursing were the only discipline consulted about a patient care problem, the range of possible solutions would be limited to nursing viewpoints and interventions. This would be simplifying the problem by categorizing it to nursing and ignoring the diversity needed from other disciplines. Problems seldom arise from just one cause, so it is ineffective to try to solve problems with just one discipline or viewpoint.

Why is reluctance to simplify challenging to healthcare organizations?

To simplify means to label or categorize to make a situation actionable. Simplification drives organization life, especially healthcare. Actions in the hospital are based on using metrics and impressions to place a situation into a known category. Reluctance to simplify is difficult, especially in healthcare, because it calls for us to suspend our beliefs and hierarchies to obtain deeper information. That deeper information is often sought in the form of multidisciplinary collaboration in which all disciplines and viewpoints are heard. True multidisciplinary collaboration remains a healthcare challenge.

What are some hospital examples of reluctance to simplify?

- A multidisciplinary group convened to address a system problem
- Root cause analysis that looks at all aspects of a system problem
- Using data as a jumping-off point to examine issues further—for example, using focus groups to dig deeper into low scores on a Patient Safety Survey
- Multidisciplinary patient care rounds with emphasis on all disciplines' participation and involvement in problem-solving

Does your work unit exhibit a reluctance to simplify? Ask:

- Is staff rewarded for asking questions, questioning the status quo, and questioning authority?
- Are people encouraged to bring up difficult problems that have the potential to stop a process or procedure?

SENSITIVITY TO OPERATIONS

What is sensitivity to operations?

Sensitivity to operations means that the organization responds and detects flaws in the system as it exists. In other words, the organization is "responsive to the messy reality" inside the system. Organizations striving for high reliability examine current processes and how real-time staff behaviors are shaped by these processes. For example, when a protocol deviation is noted, the HRO seeks to find out why the protocol was not followed rather than force a protocol that does not rationally work within the context.

Why is sensitivity to operations important to high reliability?

Sensitivity to operations concerns attention paid to how the work *is* done in real time rather than how it *should* be done. Policies, procedures, and protocols can work wonderfully on paper, but the success of these interventions is in the implementation at the work site. For example, workarounds are a symptom of an ineffective process. As workarounds persist, they become normalized, causing the system or process to become more vulnerable to failure. Sensitivity to operations detects workarounds as a symptom of impending failure to prevent this vulnerability.

Why is sensitivity to operations challenging to healthcare organizations?

Analysis of past events is the norm in the healthcare organization. Events are analyzed in terms of what should have been done dependent on existing rules or protocols. This analysis is an example of *hindsight bias*. Hindsight bias occurs when we already know the outcome and fall back on blaming the problem on user error or "this person did not follow the protocol." Hindsight bias is not helpful because it does not consider the context and why the person did a certain action. Digging deeper into the "why" is often difficult, but digging deeper unearths system causes of error that direct staff nearer to the error. Correcting these system causes is not as easy as correcting the individual, but it will lead to longer-lasting error prevention.

What are some hospital examples of sensitivity to operations?

- Examining why medications were not scanned as defined per protocol
- Examining why a rapid response team was not called when the patient met the criteria

Is your work area sensitive to operations? Ask:

- Do people doing different jobs come into enough contact with each other during the day to have a big picture of how processes are working?
- Do supervisors constantly monitor workload and throughput to ensure that resources are available for busy times or emergencies?

COMMITMENT TO RESILIENCE

What is commitment to resilience?

The Merriam Webster Dictionary defines resilience as "the ability to recover from or adjust easily to misfortune or change." The current climate of healthcare and patient care is one of change and unexpected events. Organizations that commit to resilience create an environment with resources to quickly shift gears when a change occurs so they can problem-solve, learn, and disseminate the learning and prevent further failure.

Characteristics include:

- Plan for redistributing staff for emergencies
- Ability to improvise and be creative
- Ability to form ad-hoc teams of experts

Why is commitment to resilience important to high reliability?

High reliability organizations realize that change and failures are sometimes inevitable. However, catastrophic failure can occur if organizations are not able to shift gears to constrain the damage.

Why is commitment to resilience challenging to healthcare organizations?

A main tenet of resilience is to have resources ready for surprises. Generally, organizations such as hospitals have a historic and financial mind-set of preparation for the known rather than the unknown. Preparing for the unknown requires training and preparation for emergencies and a healthy appreciation that bad things do and will happen in situations that have previously been routine.

What are some hospital examples of commitment to resilience?

- Command Center used as a vehicle for hospital collaboration for emergent events
- Immediate healthcare team collaboration or conference for changes in patient condition
- Rapid response team activation for changes in patient condition
- Debriefing of staff after unusual or rare patient care events
- Mock code blue training

Is your work area committed to resilience? Ask:

- What was the last unexpected event that occurred here? Did we have the immediate resources to problem-solve and do what was needed for the patient? Why or why not?
- What did we learn from that event? Is the learning still in practice here?

DEFERENCE TO EXPERTISE

What is deference to expertise?

Deference to expertise means that the organization allows decisions to come from people or teams from all corners of the system. Those closest to the problem are empowered to speak up and call attention to the problem and are empowered to make decisions that affect their work.

Why is deference to expertise important to high reliability?

Deference to authority, as is common in most healthcare operations, is the norm for low-risk, routine operations. However, unexpected situations often arise that the person in authority may not be in a position to recognize. Weak signals of failure are often noted by lower ranking members of the team, thus shifting the level of needed authority to those who are closest to the problem. High reliability depends on those closest to the problem to have the authority and support to speak up, make decisions, and stop a process to preserve patient safety.

Why is deference to expertise challenging to healthcare organizations?

Healthcare organizations typically and historically function in a top-down, hierarchical model, with those at the highest levels easily heard and those at the lowest levels silent. There is also a natural fear of appearing personally incompetent when acknowledging failure. Fear of reporting and structural and cultural hierarchy are two top challenges to deference to expertise.

What are some hospital examples of deference to expertise?

- Multidisciplinary timeouts prior to procedures with the ability for anyone to ask questions in a supportive environment before the start
- Multidisciplinary rounds with input from all providers and support for questions asked
- Executive rounding on nursing units for feedback
- Protocols that allow discretion and summoning of resources at the point of care: stroke protocol, RRT protocol

Does your work area defer to expertise? Ask:

- Do staff who do the work ask to be involved in decisions that affect their work?
- Do staff in this area value expertise over hierarchical rank or authority?
- Is there respect for the nature of the different jobs that people do here?

www.ingramcontent.com/pod-product-compliance
Lightning Source LLC
Chambersburg PA
CBHW051550220426
43671CB00024B/2989